Independence Day
Revolutionizing the Physician's Role in Health Care

by Richard G. Wendel, MD, MBA

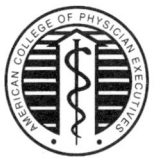

American College of Physician Executives
Suite 200
4890 West Kennedy Boulevard
Tampa, Florida 33609
813/287-2000

Copyright 2002 by the American College of Physician Executives. All rights reserved. Reproduction or translation of this book beyond that permitted by applicable copyright law without ACPE's permission is prohibited. Requests for permission to reprint or for further information should be directed to the Permissions Editor, ACPE, Suite 200, 4890 West Kennedy Boulevard, Tampa, Florida 33609.

ISBN: 0-924674-91-1
Library of Congress Card Number: 2002104263
Printed in the United States of America by A&A Printing, Tampa, FL.

Dedication

To those patients over the years who have had service complaints about my medical practice and to the practicing physicians who feel betrayed by managed care.

Preface

Physicians are disgruntled and discouraged by a medical marketplace that erodes their influence and encroaches upon their authority. Many are retiring early; others are telling their sons and daughters to pursue any career other than medicine. Intermediaries dictate policy, rules, and regulations that are increasingly intrusive to the sanctity of the doctor/patient relationship. The practicing physician feels hammered, ignored, and powerless. It's time for a physician revolution. This manuscript crafts the strategies for a successful revolt that returns the franchise back to the physician.

Physicians direct 85 percent of all expenditures on health care. This gives them the agency and the capability to appropriately channel the consumption of health care dollars. Medical practice is micro-managed, one patient at a time. This direct interface between doctor and patient has and always will appropriately form the valid definition of "managed care." This book proposes that the community of physicians supported by modern information technology has the ability to manage the patient relationship and administer the system in the most cost-effective manner without meddlesome interference from intermediaries. Physician leadership and direction is the only solution to the current crisis in health care. The alternatives are limited; more of the same fragmented managed competition or a federal single-payer system. Neither is palatable to the practicing physician.

In reviewing the literature on medical management and the medical marketplace, one is struck by the paucity of titles and books authored by physicians who have extensive experience in caring for patients. Business professionals, consultants, and academics provide the vast majority of the commentary about medicine. Perhaps practicing physicians are too busy coping with patient loads and physician executives are too preoccupied with meeting the demands of new rules and regulations. The need for greater physician involvement in transforming the medical marketplace is obvious.

Physicians often voice the opinion that the traditional institutions in organized medicine have failed and are responsible for the disenfranchisement of the physician as the pivotal player in the present medical marketplace. True, organized medicine has exhibited resistance to change, and medical practices have been slow to adopt modern business processes and newer information technology to enable efficient practice management. However, most of the systemic problems in the medical industry stem from federal government intervention. Federal programs and legislation during the past 30 years have produced excess capacity on the supply side across all health care service providers. Moreover, federal dollars have championed medical research and the introduction of expensive new technology. This excessive "supply state," coupled with increased patient demands and expectations, fosters an environment of overutilization that accounts for the rapid rise in health care costs. The system is bloated. This book identifies the elements in the system that account for the slack and suggests physician-guided solutions to contain the waste of health care dollars.

The macro-management initiatives of managed care and price competition produce few market successes and lead to many failures. Although promised, documented improvement in the quality of health care has been elusive. Moreover, managed competition produces added systemic stress on all providers while achieving only modest temporary cost control by decreasing reimbursements and limiting care. Administrative transaction costs have skyrocketed for the medical practitioner, and the inherent mutual trust embodied in the doctor-patient relationship has been undermined by third parties. Physician response is often portrayed as stemming from greed and unbridled self-interest. In reality, alien and conflicting market conditions confound and threaten the medical practitioner, who is uncertain how to respond other than with survival instincts.

Introduction

This book provides a framework for appropriate physician response to lead the change process in health care delivery and to improve the system. Its step-by-step approach to adopting strategies will empower the physician to reengineer the marketplace and regain the franchise.

This book pieces together a comprehensive plan for physicians to take charge. Chapter I outlines "patient-focused strategies" to evolve medical practices into exemplary service organizations. Chapter II focuses on ways to proactively manage the patient relationship in a medical practice. It draws heavily on new information technology (IT) that is the enabler of management through information control and patient education. Chapter III addresses waste and provides a fresh look at cost containment. Chapter IV supplies a plan that supports direct contracting by a medical group with subscriber populations. Finally, Chapter V provides a practical overview of the reengineering process.

This book is written for all physicians, physician managers, medical practice executives, and patient advocates. It offers a systemic approach to medical practice development that increases the scope of activities and features that makes the medical practice a complete integrated business entity to serve the patient and to administer health care. Through networking and collaboration, physicians have the intellectual and creative resources to effect revolutionary change in a new market environment of patient advocacy and husbanding of medical resources.

Acknowledgements

This book began as a consulting manual limited to the introduction of patient-focused strategies into medical practices. James Cummane, managing partner in the Value Creation Group in Melbourne, Australia, assisted in the patient service models.

After consulting with medical practices in the customer service area, the author soon realized that, in order to serve a greater share of the patient's health care needs, medical practices needed to actively manage the patient relationship. His work at Prophysys, Inc., a medical software company in Cincinnati, Ohio, convinced him that electronic automation offered the practicing physician the opportunity and the capability to carry out this new discipline of management. He realized that the data generated and compiled in managing the patient relationship position a medical group practice to directly contract with purchasers of health care.

The author is indebted to many professional colleagues for ideas and reviews that have improved the manuscript, given him encouragement, and prevented him from working in a vacuum. Gerald Watson, a medical software specialist, supplied the case study in Appendix C—"Dollars and Cents of an EMR." Others include John Albers, Nancy Cummane, Russell Dean, Sandy Eustis, Dan Gahl, Mike Gilligan, Sue Sherman, and Clint Schertzer.

About the Author

Dr. Wendel attended Dartmouth College and graduated from the University of Cincinnati College of Medicine. In 1997, he received an MBA from Xavier University. He is a member of Alpha Omega Alpha, Pi Kappa Epsilon, and Beta Gamma Sigma honorary societies and has authored more than a score of scientific articles. He has been active in the residency training programs in urology and family medicine at the University of Cincinnati and has been awarded the "Excellence in Teaching Award" in family medicine twice. He currently is a practice management consultant for group practices and medical software companies.

Thirty-one years as an urologist and a diverse range of activities have provided Dr. Wendel with a 360-degree perspective of the medical system and managed care. These activities include President of the Medical Staff and member of the Board of Trustees at the Deaconess Hospital in Cincinnati. He served for six years as Vice Chairman of the Board of Trustees of ChoiceCare, the largest managed care organization in Cincinnati, with a peak enrollment of 288,000. In 1968, he was Commander of a 100-bed acute care prisoner-of-war hospital in Quinhon, Viet Nam.

Medical practitioners share the adversity and depreciation of the physician's role in the medical marketplace. Using the tools provided in Independence Day, Dr. Wendel, in his first book, outlines comprehensive strategies and concrete initiatives for physicians to control their professional destiny and regain the franchise.

Dick and Ann Wendel have two grown children and reside in the Village of Mariemont in Cincinnati.

Introduction

In the margin, near Chapter III's cost awareness section, a colleague who reviewed the manuscript scrawled "Don Quixote." Indeed, putting this book together has been a journey studded with notions about an ideal world. I cover a vast array of ideas intended to help physicians critically rethink where they want to take their practices and how to get there. Is it just a fantasy that revolutionizing the physicians' role can be instrumental in returning the franchise for health care decision making back to physicians and patients? I don't believe we're tilting at windmills. I hope you'll find here a blueprint for major change that can produce very positive long-term results for your practice.

Physician focus groups that address major change in the role of the physician often produce worrisome responses. On the one hand, physicians express complacency. Their medical practices are providing them with a good living despite the hassle factors and shared adversity inherent in the current framework of managed care. The failure of the marketplace to contain costs, improve quality, and empower the patient is recognized but these are remote issues for the busy practitioner. Moreover, physicians express a lack of ability to change the system that is insidiously destroying their overall job satisfaction. These attitudes are flawed. First, there is little to be complacent about. There is widespread discontent with the system and service among consumers of health care.

| *Independence Day*

Patients want more from their doctors than just sterile medical treatment. There is urgency for physicians to critically evaluate and reinvent their practices to better serve and empower patients. Second, the physician community does have the influence, agency, and capability to capture the mandate to reengineer the system. They are far from being powerless bystanders.

This book presents five strategic imperatives that form the heart of a revolutionary change in the role of the physician.

- Patients want both high-quality medical care and service. Design and commit your practice to fulfilling both of these criteria.

- Patients want high-quality medical care and good health. Design and commit your practice to managing both of these aspects of health care.

- Patients want cost-effective health care. Design and commit your practice to micro-managing waste out of the system.

- Patients want choices and access. Design and commit your group practices to directly contract and afford patients better choices in the procurement of health care.

- The age of information technology has arrived. Use technology to increase productivity and efficiency and to support the other four strategic imperatives.

My experience has provided an opportunity to observe medicine from many vantage points. These including practicing physician, medical staff president, hospital board of trustees, vice chairman of the board of a large HMO, commander of an acute care Army hospital, academic physician, consultant, and patient. My 36 years of practice have witnessed an unprecedented period of turbulence and rapid fragmentation within a morphed medical system that still lacks direction. Physician leaders and managers must provide that direction by crafting a unified mission and staking the signposts that point the way.

Value Statement

Along with crafting a unified mission and vision, physicians must reassess and adapt the system of values in medicine to a new medical environment. The Hippocratic Oath states, "I will solemnly pledge myself to consecrate my life to the service of humanity, and the health of my patients will be my first consideration."

Both medical education and the medical environment often do not adequately support the values inherent in this critical mission. The expanding body of scientific knowledge places an increasing burden on medical schools just to cover the essentials in the armamentarium of medical treatments. Medical ethics is often a first-year "fluff" course that competes with the demanding subjects of anatomy, histology, and physiology. Medical student and residency matching programs select candidates using academic measurement. Good character and morality are assumed traits. Assessment of "people skills" such as empathy, bedside manner, ability to communicate, and caring are rarely critically evaluated. In fact, little formal instruction is given in these critical skills that underlie the art of medicine.

Similarly, little time is spent in identifying and understanding the costs of medical care, the escalation of which has had devastating systemic consequences. "Do no harm" is trumpeted into the physician's lexicon, but little critical consideration is given to cost-utility ratios and cost of quality of life years saved when new technology is introduced. Moreover, managed care initiatives to contain costs and limit covered services often manipulate the system into an unfriendly and even dangerous adversary to the consumer of health care.

Once trained and in practice, the physician is confronted with a new range of realities causing distraction from the primary mission of serving humanity. By necessity, the physician becomes a "business person" and must grapple with financial matters, partnership arrangements, and hospital politics. He or she must connect with managed care organizations (MCOs) that reimburse and offer incentives based on numbers of patients pushed through the office or hospital encounter and medical interventions. MCOs often manage the system in a way that forces the doctor to ration medical services. The value of holistic care services is only peripherally recognized, and they are usually uncompensated. Third-party payers police doctors by imposing a system of negative reinforcements. They measure their results with statistical surveys with a few parameters of medical care that rarely reflect overall quality of care. There are few positive reinforcements and little recognition for the cost-effective and caring physician who provides outstanding service.

Historically, physicians have enjoyed a high degree of autonomy and independence. When coupled with the paucity of good clean data to accurately define quality of care, this autonomy has produced a lack of standardization of medical practices, which makes measuring and documenting accountability problematic. Nevertheless, with improving statistical analysis supported by information technology, the day when a physician can explain away this issue by stating, "I cannot define quality of medical care, but I know it when I see it," is coming to an end. The privilege of autonomy must be linked to accountability.

State medical boards may sanction a physician for drug abuse, misuse of scheduled drugs, multiple catastrophic sentinel events, inappropriate sexual imposition, or lack of continuing medical education credits. However, they have not had the tools to closely monitor quality of care and intervene when a physician provides routine medical care that does not meet minimum standards.

These structural problems have allowed some bad medical practices to go unchallenged and have permitted—and even encouraged—some physicians to game the system. The author has observed a few examples of substandard medical practices that caused little notice and no action:

- A cardiologist who churned his practice by seeing patients twice a week for ECGs and PTTs.
- A generalist who fostered patient dependence by exaggerating the severity of the patient's illness.
- A surgeon who invented the scientific literature in his head and performed surgery for minimal conditions without customary indications.
- An ophthalmologist who operated on all cataracts and boasted that he made more than $2 million per year.
- A urologist who believed that radical surgery was indicated for all bladder tumors.
- An 85-year-old proctologist who declined to retire even though he had difficulty locating the operating rooms.
- An internist who was in charge of the utilization review and quality assurance committees at two hospitals for 15 years and never uncovered any instances of inferior quality of care.
- A urologist who thought only of politics and gaming the system to maximize income.

- A surgeon who did a large number of unnecessary surgeries just prior to retirement for that last transfusion of income.
- A medical staff president who abused his position by being partisan to his friends.
- A podiatrist who had an 80 percent yearly turnover rate of employees because he exhibited no concern for his office staff.
- A physician who never read a medical journal following his medical training.
- A talented surgeon who viewed his patients as numbers.
- An entrepreneurial surgeon who was interested only in the revenues his clinics generated.
- A color-blind urologist who, without supporting data, treated routine prostatosis with multiple needle aspiration.
- A radiation oncologist who never saw a consult whom he did not treat with radiation.

These are flagrant examples of substandard practice of medicine. For every marginal physician there are dozens of great physicians that practice consistently high-quality medicine. Accountability is a core value for the medical profession, and, at the end of the day, it is the physician community alone that must notice and take appropriate action.

New Trends: Cause for Optimism

Many positive trends are taking place in the marketplace that help to ensure standardization of high-quality health care:

- Medical Group formation that fosters interaction and information exchange between associates. These groups can influence utilization, produce clean data that bring to light atypical medical practices, and offer a forum for CQI.
- Standards and critical pathways crafted by a range of medical societies and organizations that support databases that enable tracking of patterns of practice and resource utilization.
- Empowerment of patients through access to information from a

variety of reliable sources so that they can participate in selecting options and making decisions in their medical care.

✦ Physician report cards generated from patient satisfaction and other surveys.

✦ Data banking and resources that permit comparison of outcomes and quality parameters.

✦ Enhanced physician capability to interact and exchange information via electronic means.

So far, we have discussed values as they relate to structural issues that affect the quality of prescriptive care in the medical system. We need to add to this value by issuing a clarion call to the physician community for a paradigm shift. Treating patients is an integral part of medical care, but it is just part of the mission. Maintaining the best possible health status and life cycle functionality for the patient is the new overriding value prescription for the physician. These initiatives include a range of health maintenance issues, such as healthy lifestyle counseling, health risk assessment and screening, continuity of care and compliance with agreed upon treatments, interaction and exchange of information, patient education, empowerment of the patient to make health care choices, and a holistic approach to the individual patient. To perform these things well is a daunting task and an unprecedented mandate for change for the practicing physician. Preventive and predictive medicine is where the action will be in the 21st Century. This paradigm shift in value has become both economically and operationally achievable for the practicing physician using the tools afforded by new electronic technology. The doctor/patient relationship and the patient relationship with a medical practice will have added importance during this transformation of medical practice. The physician and his or her practice can cope with and offer "one-stop shopping" for the health care consumer. To cement patient loyalty, medical practices will need to adopt a service ethic and new goals of health promotion to meet the needs and wants of patients. Exemplary customer service will bond the patient to your practice.

This book proposes a paradigm shift in values for a medical practice. It outlines a group of strategies for a medical practice to "be all it can be" for all patients that enter the office. "Owning" the patient's entire experience in health care is key to "owning" the marketplace. Moreover, it focuses on professionalism that leads to self-governance, self-determination, and self-policing that define Independence Day for the practicing physician. See if your practice can institutionalize some of the new value chain.

Contents

Dedication	iii
Preface	v
Acknowledgements	ix
About the Author	xi
Introduction: Physician Values	xiii

Chapter I Patient-Focused Strategies: 1
A Medical Practice Imperative
  The Cycle of Service Model 5
  The Hierarchy of Patient Value Model 8
  Value Mapping 11
  Patient Satisfaction Surveys 15
  The Office Staff: Invaluable Asset, ... 17
  Important Customer
  Another Important Customer: 19
  The Referring Doctor

Chapter II Managing the Patient Relationship: 23
Practice Excellence through Information
Exchange and Control

	The Automated "Wired" Practice:	26
	The Facilitator	
	The Return on Investment from	34
	an Electronic Office	
	Implementing the Electronic Conversion	36
	Profitable Patients	39
	Physician Stewardship:	42
	The Paradigm Shift	
	Physician Time Constraints and	44
	Reimbursements	
	The Patient Management Program	45
	The Information Asset	54
Chapter III	Controlling Healthcare Costs:	57
	A Physician's Prescription	
	Cost Awareness	59
	First Dollar Coverage	60
	Aging Populations	61
	Medical Technology	62
	Unnecessary Interventions	65
	Oversupply of Medical Providers	67
	Medical Practice Overhead	69
	MCO Administrative Expense	70
	Patient Expectations	71
	The High Cost of Dying	71
	Pharmaceuticals	73
	Health Promotion/Disease Prevention	74
	Stamping Out Disease	74
	Unwarranted Tests	75
	Treatment Venue	76
	Patterns of Practice	77
	Medical Mistakes	78
Chapter IV	Direct Contracting:	81
	Reclaiming the Franchise	
	An Administrative Model for	85
	Direct Contracting	
	Structural Requirements	87
	Operational Considerations	89
Chapter V	The Reengineering Process	93

Appendix A	Value Mapping Worksheets: .... 97 How Does Your Practice Stack Up?
Appendix B	Health Maintenance Software 129
Appendix C	Dollars and Cents of an EMR 131
Related Books	 133

Chapter 1
Patient-Focused Strategy: A Medical Practice Imperative

At the bridge table, three players discussed a local dermatologist. One had to wait six weeks to get an appointment, one was left waiting in a treatment room for 90 minutes, and one noted that the doctor had never returned his many telephone calls.

Is it surprising that two of the three had defected to other dermatologists and that none had voiced a complaint to the doctor or his staff?

Physicians are well trained to provide excellent prescriptive medical care. However, being the recipient of excellent medical care is only a part of a patient's total experience. From a patient's standpoint, there are many interactions and transactions in the process of receiving care that define a medical practice's quality of service, many of which do not directly relate to treatment of illness. Each of these service events can produce patient satisfaction or dissatisfaction. To achieve total patient satisfaction, all of the interactions, transactions, and images generated in providing care by a medical practice must be integrated to produce an *exceptional* experience for the patient.

To adopt a patient service strategy first requires a medical practice to examine the practice through the eyes of patients. The wants and needs of patients become the drivers for the design of the internal processes and procedures of a practice. In striving to be an exemplary service organization, a medical practice must make a commitment to meet and, when possible, exceed patients' expectations.

What patients consider of value is at the core of a patient-focused strategy. By producing this value, the medical practice achieves a competitive advantage when compared with other practices. The business definition of value is the summation of the benefits and sacrifices that result as a consequence of a customer's using a product or service to meet certain needs. The following value formula introduces a schematic way to view value from a patient's perspective.

VALUE = the COST (sacrifice) minus the QUALITY OF CARE (benefit) multiplied by the QUALITY OF THE EXPERIENCE

Using this equation, on what basis can physician practices gain competitive advantage?

Cost (sacrifice): In the current marketplace, medical practices do not directly compete on the cost of their services. Third-party payers fix fees. Because the vast majority of patients have insurance and medical needs are compelling, patients rarely consider cost. There is little price elasticity in medical services. Thus, in the current environment, being the low-cost physician provider does not beneficially differentiate your practice from another in the eyes of the patient.

Quality of Care (benefit): The physician community knows that wide differences exist between individual practices with regard to patterns of practice, resource consumption, and patient outcomes. Unfortunately, the patient community has no frame of reference by which to evaluate these differences. This produces an asymmetry of information between suppliers and purchasers of health care. Patients expect to receive exemplary medical care from their doctors. Quality of prescribed medical care obviously has great value, but it is usually taken for granted by the patient and usually, except by reputation, does not differentiate one medical practice from another.

Quality of the Experience (benefit): From a patient's perspective, the relationship with a practice is based on the entire experience of a visit to a physician. The service attributes of a medical practice constitute the real differences between medical practices. In the cycle of medical service, less than 10 percent of the medical visit is usually spent in face-to-face contact with the physician. The other 90 percent contributes greatly to the basis for the patient's perceptions of the medical practice. Herein lies the patient value that affords competitive advantage and, through the eyes of the patient, usually differentiates one practice from another.

This model conceptualizes value as stemming from a satisfying experience for the patient in the entire cycle of service in an episode of care. The cycle of service includes all events that highlight the encounter, including making an appointment, transportation and parking, greetings and waits, interviews, instructions, scheduling, and so on. This concept of value requires a physician to transform the medical practice to produce total patient satisfaction with each of these service events. The patient focus that is introduced has synergies with good prescriptive medical care.

Consultants offer a wide range of support services to physician practices. In most instances, these isolated silos of operational assistance are not focused primarily on providing superior service to the patient and therefore often fail to produce improved service performance. Why do consultants often avoid customer service issues? To refocus a physician's practice on service often requires change in the embedded characteristics and cultural infrastructure of a medical practice. This reengineering may carry the physician and staff outside their comfort zone. As a consequence, the consultant may be viewed as overly judgmental and intrusive, and the ensuing disruption to customary practices may result in his or her dismissal.

What should be the role of the consultant? Many define a consultant as someone who comes into your domain and asks you for your watch so that they can tell you the time. *Customer-focused* consultants step well beyond this definition. They do analyze the way things are, but, more important, they consider multiple silos that help lead their clients down the path to how things should or could be. They are change agents that seek buy-in to a new customer-focused strategy, energize the entire office staff into a team, and facilitate the gradual evolution of the practice into an exemplary service organization.

Many physicians want to be left alone to practice their brand of prescriptive medicine. However, the day when a doctor could get away with inferior service, such as long waits, limited access, and poor phone response, because of a corner on a specialty or because of supply and demand considerations is nearing an end. Today's market and health consumer demand much more. The wise physician should listen to the message and not kill the messenger.

Figure 1-1.

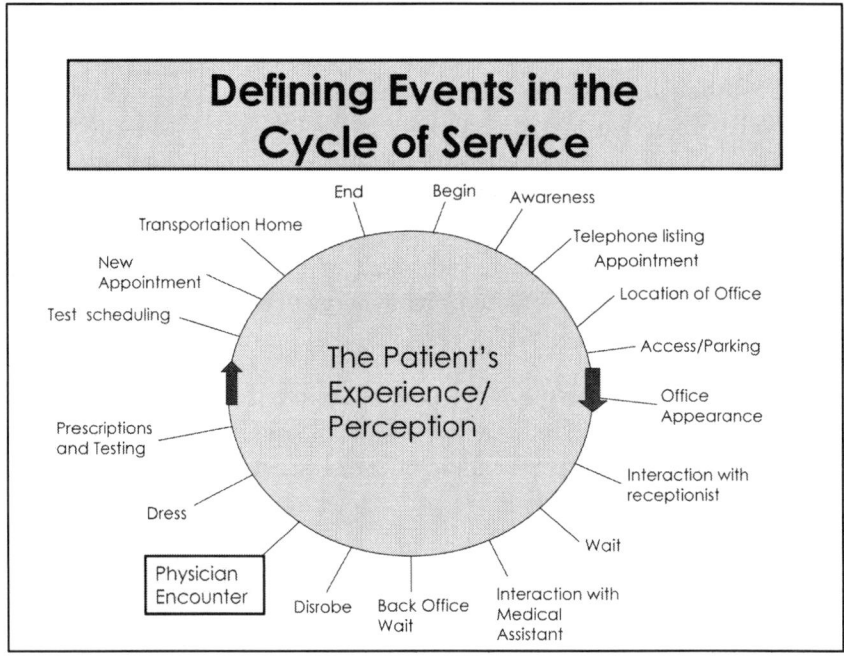

The benefits to a medical practice that accrue from a shift to a patient-focused strategy are compelling. Practice volume and associated revenues increase because of higher rates of patient retention, return, and referrals. The increased trust and comfort level improves patient compliance with treatment. Office expense decreases or remains unchanged because of the lower transaction costs derived from loyal patients. Employee satisfaction and recognition increase with the positive feedback received from satisfied patients.

In summary, providing a completely satisfying experience to the patient holds the key to a successful medical practice. Designing the processes and procedures in a medical *practice to delight* and exceed the patient's expectations cements patient satisfaction and loyalty. This new strategy expands and builds on the traditional doctor/patient relationship. To implement the shift to a patient focus requires physicians to analyze their practices with new metrics of service excellence.

The Cycle of Service Model: Understanding the Patient Experience

The first conceptual model, the Cycle of Service Model, assists in understanding the total experience through the eyes of the patient. This model breaks down the patient experience into *defining events or moments of truth* that highlight the episode of care (figure 1-1, page 4). When the episode of care is compartmentalized, the attributes of each defining event can be evaluated from a patient's perspective. Patient feedback then forms the basis for service quality improvements.

Sampling of Events That Contribute to the Patient Experience

First introduction to the medical practice:

✦ Patient, friend, co-worker, or physician testimonial or referral

- The yellow pages, web pages
- Street signage and/or advertisement
- HMO lists of provider
- Hospital or academy of medicine referral service

✦ Office locations:

- Convenience
- Security
- Parking and transportation access
- Accommodation for the disabled

✦ Making appointments:

- Phone access
- Convenient appointment time
- Phone greeting, scheduling, and instructions
- Evening and weekend office hours

✦ Waiting room stay:

- Interaction with receptionist
- Ambience of the front office
- Reading and educational materials in the waiting room
- The wait to be called back
- Greeting from the medical assistant
- Filling out of history, insurance, and personal information forms
- Play things to amuse and occupy children during the wait

- Treatment room stay:
    - History taking and recording of vital signs by medical assistant
    - Privacy concerns
    - Courtesy of personnel
    - Chaperones
    - Layout and cleanliness of treatment rooms
    - Waiting time
    - Instructional and reading materials in treatment rooms
- Physician encounter:
    - Physician's social skills; personality, warmth, and active listening
    - Laying on of hands
    - Communication of findings, outline of treatment plans, and instructions
    - Prescriptions
    - Explanation of tests
    - Time for questions
    - Physician reassurance
    - Need for follow up
- Scheduling of tests/referrals:
    - Making arrangements
    - Referral to specialists and testing facilities
    - Verbal instructions
    - Printed instructions
- Departure:
    - Final inquiry to see if instructions were understood
    - Follow-up appointment scheduling
    - Explanation of the bill and collection of copayments
    - Transportation home
- Feedback:
    - Telephone questions
    - Retrieving lab results
    - On-line interactions

The initial defining event that results in an appointment to see a particular physician will vary from patient to patient. One patient may consider a convenient office location that was discovered in the yellow pages as the method of choosing a physician. Another may make an appointment because he or she has heard that the physician runs on schedule with short waiting times or that the office handles all insurance matters. Still others are attracted because of testimonials from friends, relatives, co-workers, or doctors; ease of making an appointment; or finding the doctor on the list of HMO providers. Hospital referral services and other agencies may also serve to introduce a patient to a physician's practice.

After making the choice of physician, each patient then enters the cycle of *defining events* in the encounter. Each *defining* event represents an interface with the practice from which the patient develops a perception of the physician's practice. In the composite, this creates the total patient experience that is the basis for patient satisfaction. The *defining* events form a value chain of service. They involve receiving information about the doctor and staff and interaction or transactions with the doctor and the staff. Each step in the flow sequence can be a source of patient discontent if the patient's expectations are not met.

Few medical practices have a thorough understanding of how their patients view the service they provide. Studies of patient satisfaction have shown that physicians usually overestimate the quality of their service, whereas office staff often underestimates the quality. An explanation for this discrepancy relates to the fact that complaints are more frequently voiced to staff members. Moreover, patients are reluctant to complain to physicians for fear of retaliation when they are vulnerable in the treatment setting. Often, reticent patient dissatisfaction translates into non-compliance with treatment, failure to follow up, and defections to other practices. Feedback tactics to increase the percentage of complaints that are heard are an important part of all patient-focused strategies.

Patients' needs and wants will vary. Some may consider the length of waiting time a defining event whereas others may enjoy sitting in the waiting room reading magazines. Some patients may prefer casual informality, with the use of first names, while other may prefer to be addressed in a more formal manner. Individual preferences may make some service attributes unimportant or neutral with regard to either building or undermining patients' experiences. It is essential that a practice understand what a specific patient considers of value. Active solicitation of feedback from the patient is central to this process.

Figure 1-2.

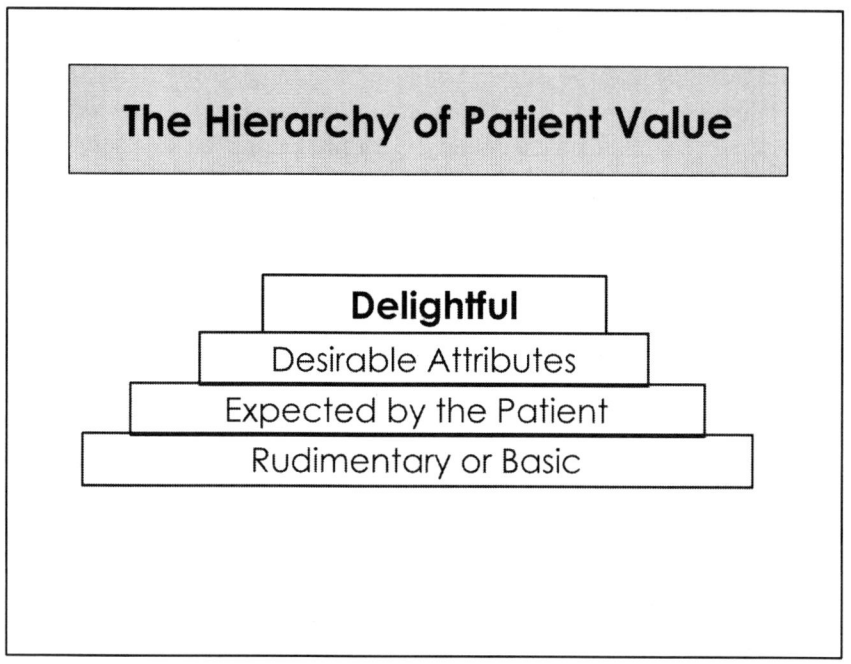

Patient value and satisfaction are achieved by designing into each *defining event* superior service features that meet and exceed the expectations of the patient. The patient can be the best and most reliable ally the physician has in the current marketplace. Why not build your practice around providing a totally satisfying experience?

The Hierarchy of Patient Value Model: Using Creativity to Exceed the Expectations of the Patient

The Hierarchy of Patient Value Model is an additional tool to further understand, quantify, and define patient value. The model breaks down the service features of a medical practice into four levels of value. These four building blocks, Rudimentary, Expected, Desirable, and Delightful, form a pyramid of ascending value (figure 1-2, above).

Rudimentary: The lowest level comprises the basic necessities to function as a medical practice. They include an office, phone, exam room, assistant, and medical record.

The Expected: The second level includes features that are taken for granted by the patient. They are the staples of an average practice. Included in this level is a division between the front and the back office, with separation of administrative and professional activities. The physician participates in the health plan in which the patient is enrolled. Patients are able to make timely appointments, and 24-hour phone response is provided. There is a process for billing, filing insurances, communicating test results, maintaining records, and giving instructions. Confidentiality is maintained. *The patient expects the physician to be competent and exhibit professional behavior. Good prescriptive medical care is expected.* All medical practices must offer these features to compete and survive.

Desirable: Stepping up the pyramid in patient value is the desired features and attributes of a medical practice. These sets of measures and criteria elevate the medical practice above the ordinary and produce a high level of patient satisfaction. They include capable office staff members who demonstrate proficiency in their jobs. The office is comfortable, handles all insurance matters, and offers appointments for pressing problems within three days. Office hours include some evening or Saturday times. The periodicals in the waiting room are current, and waiting times are less than 30 minutes. Telephone calls are returned promptly, and there is a quick turnaround response to patient complaints. Educational materials are provided, and patients are given complete instructions and information about their conditions. Referral letters are sent by the physician to referring doctors. Office policies and procedures and information about the practice are provided to patients in a well-crafted office brochure.

These features meet the needs and wants of most patients and produce high scores for a medical practice on patient satisfaction surveys. The desirable level of patient value, however, usually does not aspire to exceed the expectations of the patient. Consequently, high satisfaction ratings often do not translate into avid patient loyalty. The recipient of this level of service may still switch physicians for reasons such as a lower premium from competing health plans, geographical factors, a preference for a hospital where the physician does not have privileges, or other personal considerations.

Delightful: This is the highest level of patient value. The features on this menu customize the patient experience. They are the most powerful factors in bonding a patient to a medical practice.

To reach this level requires creativity, a keen sensitivity to the quality of the patient experience, and a committed team approach to providing exemplary service. At this level, a medical practice continuously invents innovative ways to provide personalized service features that exceed the expectations of the patient.

Several examples can serve to illustrate outstanding personalized service. In one office the author visited, the receptionist had deftly developed her own patient following through the use of fine interpersonal skills. She remembered names, showed interest in the family events of patients, projected humor and spirit, and walked the extra mile to help patients. Her friendly demeanor highlighted the patient's experience.

One receptionist recorded where patients sit in the waiting room after check in. She shared this information with the medical assistant who could then approach the patient with direct eye contact using a low tone of voice to call them back. The patients felt they were more than a number.

One office provides a telephone for local calls. During the wait, the patient is offered coffee and is invited to view educational videos on health-related subjects.

Many outstanding practices target minimal or no waiting time and office appointments that can be scheduled on the same day an urgent request to see the doctor is received. An array of teaching videos and printed instructions can be used to educate and inform patients. Mailings of health promotional materials that answer frequently asked questions and assist the patient with decision making are a reminder that the doctor cares. The presence of a graduate nurse or nurse practitioner projects a professional image and adds intellectual capital that complements the medical skills and efficiency of the physician. Giving free samples to the patient to start treatment and offering free screening tests that are often unexpected fosters patient rapport and loyalty.

If patients are to be referred, a call by the doctor or a staff member to schedule the appointment and provide pertinent information is often unanticipated. This process improves compliance, obtains an expedient appointment, and decreases the burden on the patient. Personalized letters sent to the patient after an initial or annual general physical that detail the results of the visit and laboratory values can be powerful instruments to please, congratulate, and reassure.

Figure 1-3.

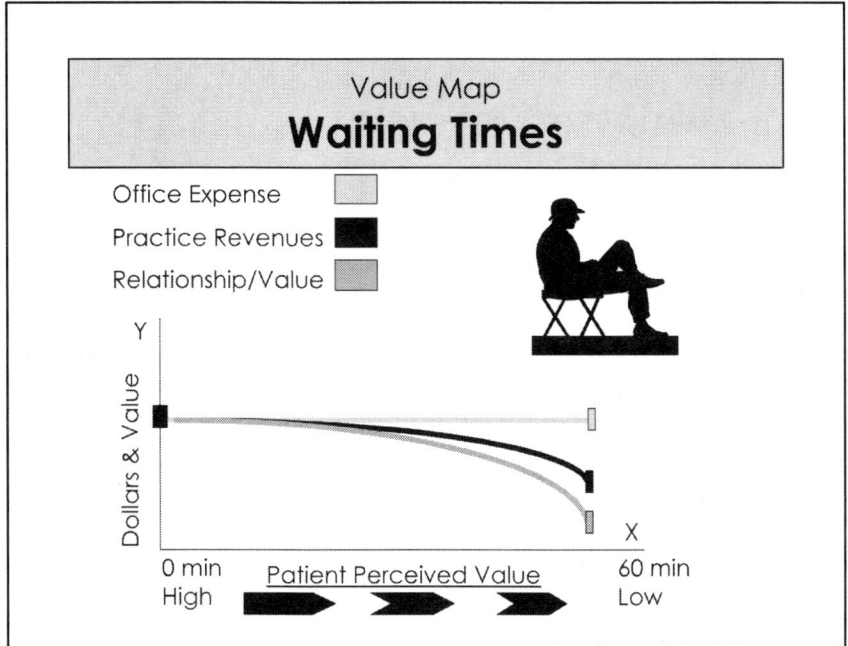

Thank you cards for patient referrals delight the patient who made the referral. It adds a personal touch.

A dressing cubicle in the treatment room to afford complete privacy when the patient is undressing or dressing is welcomed. Examination gowns that cover the body can help to minimize the embarrassment of the visit.

These are just a representative group from myriad innovative ways to exceed the expectations of the patient. In a medical practice, these finely tuned amenities provide the real substance that translates into patient value and loyalty.

Value Mapping: A Model for Quality Service Improvement for a Medical Practice

Value Mapping offers one approach to dissecting and breaking down the service attributes and features of a medical practice. It offers a framework for continuous quality service improvement.

In the Value Mapping Model, the service features and attributes of a medical practice are analyzed from five perspectives:

1. The patient's perspective
2. How to detect whether a problem exists
3. The root causes of the problem
4. Solutions
5. Cost considerations

After an identified problem has been dissected, a value map can be constructed that depicts the impact on a medical practice of a service deficiency. The graph plots office expense, revenue generation, and relationship value on the y-axis, and the perceived patient value and parameter measure to be evaluated on the x-axis. Using best practice benchmarks, service quality improvements can be monitored and measured. We will use waiting times to illustrate the process (figure 1-3, page 11).

Patient Perspective:

Long waiting times are by far the most common patient complaints that cause dissatisfaction and defections. Patients increasingly expect to be seen at their scheduled appointment times and become resentful when not seen on time. How often have you heard a patient say about a doctor, "He's a good doctor, but he is always late?" To be patient-focused, a physician must believe that a patient's time is as valuable as his or her own.

Most established patient visits consume a predictable amount of the physician's time. Running behind in the schedule does not alter the workload; it only causes displeasure and inconvenience for patients. No matter how understanding of the physician's time constraints the patient is, consistently long waiting times send a message that the doctor just doesn't care.

How to Detect a Problem:

A problem with waiting times is easily uncovered. Ask the office staff; they receive immediate feedback from dissatisfied patients. Likewise, it is the perennial sore spot detected in patient satisfaction surveys that permit simple measurement.

Root Causes for the Problem:

Sometimes the cause may not be obvious.

✦ Usually the finger is pointed at the doctor, who uses an arsenal of excuses to explain the tardiness. A pattern of being chronically late usually reflects character traits.

✦ A flawed scheduling process.

✦ Inexperienced scheduling personnel, which often reflects a high employee turnover rate.

✦ Staff or physician manipulation of the schedule to meet personal needs.

✦ Interruption of office hours by outside activities.

✦ Inefficiency and lack of motivation.

Solutions:

Decreasing waiting times requires change in patterns of behavior that are often deeply embedded in the culture of an office practice. If a medical practice can pursue one or more of the following steps and measure the results, the benefits from a culture of punctuality can be appreciated. The doctor must understand that a problem exists and want to take positive steps to address it:

✦ Get the office force involved in seeking a solution to the problem. The staff usually has many constructive and insightful ideas.

✦ Examine the scheduling process and time allotments.

✦ Train the scheduling personnel.

✦ Expand office hours if necessary.

✦ Set a benchmark goal of making waiting times less than 15 minutes.

✦ Periodically measure waiting times, and solicit patient feedback to assess improvement.

✦ Simple tactics to afford flexibility in the schedule.

  – Leave an hour gap late in the schedule to work in urgent and emergency patients. This decreases the number of phone calls that require immediate attention from the doctor and emergency department visits.

– Have a dedicated time for brief encounters, such as routine BP checks, simple suture removal, or adjustment of medication.

✦ Take steps to improve the experience of waiting.

– Notify the patient if the doctor is significantly behind, and give him or her the opportunity to arrive later or reschedule.

– Notify waiting patients at 10-15 minute intervals about how much further delay to expect and assure them they have not been forgotten.

– Have a telephone in the waiting room, provide coffee and spring water, show educational videos about health matters, provide an assortment of current periodicals, and have children's books and play things available.

Cost Considerations:

When a doctor consistently runs late, it raises the transaction costs of doing business and decreases practice revenues. Why?

✦ Patients badger the receptionist.

✦ Patients may walk out, reschedule, criticize your practice to their friends, and defect.

✦ The doctor and staff have to spend more time to overcompensate and effect a turnaround.

✦ Patients may choose not to keep follow-up appointments.

✦ Transaction costs of rescheduling are increased.

To be on time *delights* most patients, plus it creates harmony and decreases tension in the office. Decreases in waiting and cycle time are linked to increased staff productivity, increased patient satisfaction, increased revenues, and decreased office expense. Punctuality is a pure positive reinforcing behavior.

In consulting, a variety of value maps can be utilized. These include service features such as convenient appointments, phone response, communications, privacy, bedside manner, and so on. (See Appendix A: Value Mapping Worksheets: How Does Your Practice Stack Up?) From this composite picture, we identify and address areas in need of improvement. Targeted measures are crafted collaboratively, and a program for service excellence is initiated. Success hinges on physician and staff commitment to the change process.

Patient Satisfaction Surveys: Discovering the Service Features Your Patients Value

The majority of medical practices do not have an ongoing program to collect and track patient satisfaction information derived from surveys or interactions with patients. Without a systematic program to actively solicit feedback from patients, a medical practice is handicapped in any effort to identify and resolve complaints or to improve service features that are valued by patients.

In most practices, there is ample discussion of the occasional unhappy patient who voices dissatisfaction, disrupts normal operations, harasses the staff, and threatens to defect. Informal discussion among staff members of these events does not provide a comprehensive assessment of the service attributes in a medical practice.

The subjective perceptions of the physician and the staff about the quality of service often do not correlate with patient value, or with measured patient satisfaction scores.

It is generally conceded that about 95 percent of all patient complaints are never expressed or brought to the attention of a medical practice. On the other hand, the medical practice can be certain that the unhappy patient's grapevine of friends will hear the complaint. Many reasons account for this reluctance to directly criticize a medical practice, including no one cares, it's not worth the effort, and the patient does not know to whom to complain. Additionally, the patient may feel vulnerable to retaliation if he or she voices a complaint to the doctor who is entrusted with his or her personal medical care.

An embedded program to uncover patient dissatisfaction and to actively listen to patients provides substantial benefits for a medical practice. For instance, a number of studies have shown that timely turnaround of complaints in most instances results in retention of dissatisfied patients and enhances patient loyalty. Understanding the patient with unmet expectations provides the practice with the opportunity to formulate a set of activities that correct service deficiencies and produce patient value.

Patient satisfaction surveys provide a convenient method to affordably evaluate patient satisfaction. Patients have a high degree of emotional involvement and attachment to their doctors, and most patients are agreeable to completing confidential patient satisfaction surveys.

Patient satisfaction surveys can be crafted to answer virtually any service question. The questionnaire should be brief and the questions objective, specific, and scaled. An occasional global or open-ended question that permits the patient to voice individual concerns can be revealing. Standardization of surveys used in practices is desirable to permit practice comparisons and to quantify interval improvement results. To increase the number of surveys completed and returned, have patients address the envelope in which they receive the survey after the visit. This gives them a feeling of participation. Additionally, front office staff can be trained to subtly measure satisfaction by discussing service issues with the family and attendants of the patient. Another tactic to generate patient feedback includes an old-fashioned suggestion box positioned under a sign; *Your Comments Help Us Improve Our Service.*

Analysis of patient satisfaction studies reveals generally higher scores in populations over the age of 50, lower in practices with greater than 10 doctors, and lower in patient groups enrolled in HMO and PPO health care products.

In addition to patient satisfaction surveys, two other tracking initiatives are useful in taking the service pulse of a medical practice. The first quantifies the number of patients who defect to other practitioners. Exit interviews can be used to understand why a patient leaves your practice. This may elucidate breakdowns in the service experience and serve as a guide for your service improvement program.

The second tracks the number of new patients seen month to month. This can be converted to graph form and displayed as a measure of practice growth. It is also useful to track the numbers of referrals broken down by doctors, friends, relatives and so on. Both defector interviews and new patient win rates incur little expense and effort to track and record.

The higher the quality of the data and measures that exist to portray the service pulse of a practice, the better equipped a practice is to take corrective measures to solve problems in customer service. Measurement is a critical component of any service improvement process. The more you know, the more able you are to serve.

All survey instruments introduce problems with population sampling, response rates, design, and objectivity. But, in a medical practice, the tabulated results and validity are probably of less importance than the process. The process brings into focus and stimulates dialog among employees about patient service issues.

One final caveat: Patient satisfaction surveys measure satisfaction and dissatisfaction and do not always correlate in a linear fashion with patient loyalty. Loyalty is more difficult to measure and more directly relates to a satisfying experience that fulfills the service criteria that the individual patient considers important. One patient may equate value to a close relationship with the physician, whereas another may consider minimal waiting times and convenience the signature features that produce value. On surveys, questions that quantify what circumstances might cause the patient to switch doctors and whether the patient would refer friends and relatives can give clues to the degree of patient loyalty.

The Office Staff: Invaluable Asset, Important Customer

Many activities of the office staff add value to the patient's experience. However, many routine activities, such as chart filing, procurement of supplies, addressing envelopes, bill paying, and maintaining files, have little direct relationship to the provision of service to the patient. These essential repetitive chores are the mundane realities of office work.

To counterbalance these monotonous tasks, employees need the motivation derived from a purposeful mission of service. Providing a totally satisfying experience for the patient provides that stimulus. All studies support the observation that the job satisfaction ratings of office employees always mirror the level of patient satisfaction enjoyed by a medical practice.

Employees are the internal customers of a physician's practice and a highly prized asset that needs continuous cultivation. Doctors are often only peripherally aware of how the work gets done in the office to support normal operations. A common complaint voiced by employees is "the doctor never says thank you or shows appreciation." Encouragement, appreciation, or simple acknowledgement of a job well done motivates and energizes the staff.

If a physician wants a high performance office force, he or she must supply the guidance for its formation. Leadership characteristics that support office team behavior include fairness, consistency, consideration, and participation. Experience shows that, even without these leadership qualities, the office force will still show loyalty to the physician who is friendly, interactive, and provides good prescriptive medical care.

Selective recruitment, thorough training, and a learning team are the three building blocks that afford the staff infrastructure for a practice to excel and become an exemplary service organization.

Recruitment: Office personnel are the direct representatives and agents of the doctor. Nothing is more critical to a practice than hiring employees with the requisite skills and the aptitude to work in a "people environment" that requires emotional stability and empathy. A dedicated due diligence process helps to overcome the many pitfalls of hiring and satisfactorily filling vacancies. Being very selective in hiring pays dividends that more than make up for the added expense and transaction time. High employee turnover rates can be devastating to a medical practice. It is estimated that turnover of one employee costs the business the equivalent of 18 months' salary.

Training: Few medical practices have a formal training program for staff. On-the-job training is often the only type of learning experience. Often, employees are plugged into jobs without specialized training, and job responsibilities are horizontally and vertically expanded arbitrarily. Empowerment boundaries and ownership of specific functions are poorly defined. A consultant often hears complaints about initial and subsequent training received by the staff.

An office force that has the necessary skills, knowledge, and abilities to master office functions, work efficiently together, and focus on serving the patient enhances practice success. A high performance staff makes the physician's life less complicated and minimizes the "hassle factor" in medical practice. Additionally, high-quality employees facilitate further recruitment and make the physician's office a good place to work. Adequate training opportunities motivate an office staff and send a signal that the physician cares about employees. The intellectual capital that stems from thorough training far overshadows the costs.

Learning Team: The best office forces work as committed teams. They are a functional family that continuously models a rich and efficient office culture. Because the physician is usually focused on the professional component of service and not the business of medicine, the staff of a medical practice enjoys a degree of autonomy and self-direction that is seldom seen in other large or small businesses. Thus, a self-directed team approach that feeds on interaction, cooperation, and caring should be cultivated and encouraged. Physicians should empower their employees to take initiative, solve problems, and think independently.

The term "office culture" is difficult to accurately define. An organization's culture encompasses both the overt or conscious and covert or subconscious environment in the medical office. If harmony and competence characterize an office culture, it produces the glue and matrix upon which to build a high performance team. The physician is the enabler, facilitator, and steward of office culture. He or she shoulders the responsibility for setting the stage. If the culture is overt and mature, it blossoms and can be a great source of satisfaction, support, and enhanced productivity for the doctor. This in turn creates an environment that can produce a totally satisfying experience for the patient when he or she visits the doctor.

Another Important Customer: the Referring Doctor

Primary care doctors and specialists often appear to be in separate, opposing camps. Many factors contribute to this division. Gatekeeping in managed care has vested increased power and control with PCPs. The ongoing, heated debate over direct patient access to specialty care attests to the gravity of this issue. Invasive testing and surgical procedures are compensated at higher relative values than office visits. As a result, there are disparities in incomes between PCPs and specialists that are often a source of resentment. Generally, surgeons and generalists are different personality types. Office practice provides the majority of revenues for a PCP, whereas for most specialists it affords just enough revenue to pay office expenses. The income of a specialist is usually linked to the number of procedures performed. Often, PCPs feel there is little need to actively communicate patient information to specialists, and specialists in turn refer to other physicians without consulting with the PCP. Moreover, both PCPs and specialists have many subtle misconceptions about each other. Despite these tensions, the differences must be bridged and a cooperative relationship forged to afford comprehensive, seamless medical care.

Referral patterns are often perceived as being driven by friendship, peer groups, politics, entertaining, and affability. These collegial factors are important, but experience reveals that, the majority of the time, loyal referral patterns and relationships between PCPs and specialists develop from open communication, availability, and courtesy. They are the cornerstones of building a practice from physician referrals and are essential for both PCP and specialists.

Open Communication Practices that Enhance the Relationship

- Timely, personalized thank you referral letters that contain essential information. If a PCP sends a referral letter to a specialist, it is guaranteed to exceed expectations and be remembered.

- A short note or brief telephone call from the PCP to introduce a new patient referral to the specialist is always appreciated.

- Periodic contact from the specialist to keep the PCP informed about a patient's course of treatment and progress.

- PCP and specialist interactively participating in scientific sessions and committee work at the hospital.

- Get to know your colleagues by working the doctor's lounge; take the initiative to introduce yourself and develop a first name relationship.

- Be engaging on a personal basis; avoid discussing just the doom and gloom in the medical marketplace and focus on the other physician's interests.

- Be a good listener.

- Inform referring physicians about newer techniques, treatments, and services that you offer.

- Attend hospital staff meetings and functions at your primary hospitals.

- Dress appropriately to communicate a professional image; save sneakers, sport shirts, and sloppy dress for sporting events.

- Hospital nurses play a vital role in the chain of communication among doctors. Keep them informed and view them as customers; they are often asked for opinions in the selection of a doctor.

- Share with your colleagues practice strategies that have produced results.

- Generously provide "curb stone assistance" to other practitioners.

Availability

- Use electronic technology to be reachable 24 hours a day; use cell phones, beepers, and newer devices such as web-enabled PDAs.
- Hire a responsive answering service or maintain a call center that can prioritize calls and reach you.
- Provide after-hour coverage by responsive physicians with equivalent backgrounds.
- Make hospital rounds in the morning when there is the greatest traffic of other doctors making rounds.
- See referred patients in the office or hospital as soon as possible, and immediately call the referring doctor after seeing a patient.
- Call the referring doctor whenever surgery or testing is scheduled on an emergency basis.
- Do not treat serious problems involving new patients in the hospital by phone at night; make the run to the hospital. Let the referring doctor know of your concern for the patient.
- Be available to see consults over holidays and weekends.
- Participate in the emergency department on-call schedule.
- Place a higher priority on the patient's comfort and well-being than on your social calendar.
- Creatively use electronic technology to permit open connectivity with referring physicians.

Courtesy

- Never direct patients away from referring physician unless there are compelling quality issues.
- Never refer patients to other doctors without knowledge and approval of referring physician.
- Never openly criticize referring physician.
- If possible, always send referred patient to the testing facilities and hospitals used by referring physician.

- Be sensitive to risk management issues in the referral network.

- When appropriate, offer positive testimonials on the quality of care provided by the referring physician to the patient and hospital staff.

- If possible, avoid sharing the ultimate responsibility for a patient's care with another physician; try, when possible, to define the boundaries of responsibility.

Good communication skills, exceptional availability, and courtesy are essential to building a practice's referral base. In the author's experience, social activities, sporting events, playing politics, and small gratuities are less important in the larger perspective. There is no substitute for the dedication and hard work that provides service and value to the referring doctor as well as to the patient.

Summary

If a medical practice focuses on the customer and provides exemplary patient value, all measures of practice success will improve. Referral and recruitment of new patients will increase, and a higher percentage of old patients will be retained. The doctor's reputation will be enhanced. Loyal patients augment practice revenues that increase the worth and monetary value of the practice.

As larger medical groups coalesce, the success and growth of a patient-focused practice positions it well to negotiate satisfactory agreements. Loyal patients, when mobilized, can shield a practice from exclusion from HMO products.

In a marketplace with an excess number of physicians, declining reimbursements for medical services, and constant upheaval, a customer-focused practice helps to ensure survivability. Efficient practices with loyal patients should withstand any outside threat or insult.

The new paradigm requires that physicians lead and manage their organizations by refocusing their services on patients' experiences. The patient will ultimately determine the directions of medicine. Who better than the patient to have as a disciple and advocate for the physician?

Chapter 2

Managing the Patient Relationship: Practice Excellence through Information Exchange and Control

"I see my physician when I am sick. He tells me to call or return if I am having problems. My chiropractor sees me regularly for back pain. He has prescribed massage therapy, placed me on nutritional supplements, and suggested I see a naturopathic doctor. At the last visit, he gave me a pamphlet about the consequences of smoking and discussed using acupuncture to cure my smoking habit."

Who is managing this patient's health care?

The past two decades have seen physicians' commanding role in the medical environment erode. Well-capitalized managed care organizations (MCOs) and the federal Centers for Medicare and Medicaid Services (CMS), have emerged as administrators and intermediaries interposed between the physician and the patient. Their goals are to manage patient populations and medical care, and in the process they subordinate and neutralize the physician's influence.

On average administrative and marketing activities of MCOs consume between 20 and 25 percent of health care premium dollars and impose requirements on medical practices that add to the administrative and transactional costs of practicing medicine. MCOs' ever-changing and often arbitrary policies are in large measure responsible for the heightened "hassle factor" experienced by the practicing physician.

Additionally, hospitals, with their large "war chests" of retained earnings and tiers of administrators, have frantically expanded their scope of services. Often they own and administer large physician group practices that directly compete with the private practice sector. To expand revenues and capture market share, they venture beyond inpatient treatment facilities into areas such as fitness centers, sport medicine facilities, nursing homes, home health, and a wide range of specialized clinics. They covet a larger role in managing the medical marketplace. Moreover, the entrepreneurial activities of these often tax-exempt institutions have added greatly to the excess supply side of the service equation.

The fragmented physician community of traditionally small medical practices has lacked the consolidated financial resources, business acumen, and unified mission to counter these developments. In this reshuffling of the medical environment, the physician's fidelity and moral responsibility to his patients have become compromised by intermediaries that have crafted a web of competing obligations and conflicting interests. Moreover, these aggressive players have pushed the patient out of the loop of decision making and confronted them with an increasingly convoluted medical system that is often unresponsive to their needs.

To regain the franchise, physicians must manage the full scope of their patients' needs. The following chapters detail management strategies to rebalance the medical landscape by empowering physician direction and transformation and, in the process, transfer greater control to patients. Physician leadership and management offers the brightest prospect for constructive reengineering to manage costs and eliminate waste, improve the health care delivery system, and refocus on health promotion through management of the patient relationship. These strategies would curtail the influence of the intermediary "organizers" of health care. Additionally, hospitals are relegated to inpatient treatment facilities and appropriately viewed as "cost centers."

To build on the service infrastructure laid out in chapter I, we can now expand to focus proactively on managing the patient relationship. This is an active process and carries us beyond the platform of exemplary service to interactive patient advocacy. This places the physician in an expanded role as a steward, guide, and coach to enable the patient to maintain the best possible health. In this context, patient advocacy derives from an "interactive partnership" in health care between the medical practice and the patient. A range of new activities in the medical practice is crafted to produce a seamless relationship with a steady flow of information to and from the patient. Standard prescriptive medical care is supplemented with programs to support wellness initiatives and manage the full range of health-related issues. Predictive and preventive medicine is stressed, and optimal life cycle functionality of the patient becomes the primary objective. The medical practice strives to own a larger share of the patient's entire health care experience.

This management discipline takes the physician's role beyond the doctor/patient encounter in the office and hospital into the arena where the practice manages the majority of the total wellness needs of the patient. The ultimate goal is greater positive physician influence over a patient's complete life cycle of health.

The goal of capturing and "owning" the customer's total experience in purchasing and using a product or service is a contemporary business concept. The exclusive relationship that results from achievement of this goal produces the returns that enable a business to profitably and actively manage the customer relationship. By meeting the customer's full range of needs, the business is rewarded with repeat and expanded purchases, solidified customer loyalty, enhanced referrals, improved outcomes, greater customer feedback for service improvement, and the opportunity to educate and inform the customer. Management of the relationship advantageously positions the firm or practice to receive the lifetime value of a loyal customer. This concept can be applied to virtually all markets, including the medical marketplace. Electronic technology makes this goal achievable and economical.

Group practice data banks and information control, plus open connectivity afforded by information technology, offer medical groups and networks of physician groups the opportunity and capability to position themselves to provide the administrative and interactive functions necessary to:

✦ Organize and manage information about populations of patients and directly contract successfully with purchasers of health care.

✦ Collaborate and compete to eliminate unnecessary layers of intermediaries.

✦ Use information to improve quality of care.

✦ Identify and eliminate waste to contain costs.

✦ Individually manage each practice/patient relationship.

The strategy institutionalizes the physician as the driver of revolutionary marketplace change.

When discussing this new discipline of management, physicians often respond by stating emphatically that their practices already provide for these supporting activities to manage the patient relationship. If this is so, why are the majority of Americans dissatisfied with the current delivery of health care? Why do the number of office visits to other health care professionals, such as chiropractors and homeopaths, exceed those to registered physicians in the United States? Why is alternative and complementary medicine, such as acupuncture, homeopathy, massage therapy, hypnotherapy, spiritual healing, aroma, and nutritional therapy, so appealing to the well-educated consumer with chronic conditions? Why do unproven remedies and exotic treatments survive in the marketplace? The answer, in part, rests with the physician's focus on curative treatment of definable conditions. The busy physician is often distracted from the mind-body connection and the holistic needs of the patient. Physicians manage illness but do not proactively manage patient relationships. Patients have a wide range of individual medical needs; traditional treatment may head the list, but it is a long list. Physician groups must seek to become the sole resource that meets the entire health care needs and wants of patients.

In capsule form, table 2-1, page 27, summarizes the physician's changing orientation and behaviors when managing the patient relationship. The six bulleted items characterize the paradigm shift from the traditional to the transformed role of the physician. Refer to these central themes that comprise the new metrics for medical care excellence as you move through the chapter.

The Automated 'Wired' Practice: The Facilitator

Information technology plays a critical role in supporting transformational activities. First, consider any contemporary consumer Web site that strives to own the customer's total experience. The Web pages offer colorful brochureware that defines the product or service and describes its distinguishing features and benefits. They give information about the company, including mission statements, employee qualifications, policies and procedures, and convenience. Hyperlinks to other pertinent resources are provided to educate and inform the customer. Testimonials from satisfied customers reassure the customer. A shopping basket for

Table 2-1. Physician Management Change Focus

Old	New
Reactive Management	Proactive Management
Treatment	Life Cycle Functionality
Disease Management	Holistic Approach
Physician Control	Partnership in Health
Authoritative Role	Steward, Educator, Cheerleader
Patient Dependence	Patient Empowerment

easy online purchase expedites the transaction, completed with a few clicks of the mouse. Return e-mail confirms the order, and the customer can access his or her account to determine the status of the order and when it will be delivered. Warranty and service guarantees are included, with a channel for complaints and customer feedback by e-mail, snail mail, or telephone. A community chat room is offered to discuss the features of the product or service and troubleshoot problems. Passwords, encryption, and firewalls ensure the security of the transactions. The information provided in registration plus purchasing behavior by the customer guides the company to tailor its offerings to meet specific needs and wants of the customer. This customer profiling enables the company to call attention to additional products and services. E-commerce sites empower customers to shop at their convenience, 24 hours a day, and provide direct links to appropriate informational databases and resources at the touch of a finger.

Web shopping is a win-win proposition. The company saves money in transaction and in plant and equipment costs. Automated consumer response and feedback aids inventory control and supports just-in-time manufacturing. Intermediary non-value-added expense is minimized or eliminated. The customer has the ultimate convenience and efficiency of shopping at home, researching the marketplace, and making informed purchase decisions. This example of tactics used by e-commerce to own the customer's entire experience has parallels to a medical practice managing the patient relationship.

Today, an expanding number of dot-com companies are producing well-advertised medical Web sites that offer an extensive menu of information and resources. It would seem unlikely that these large national and international Web sites will meet the needs of local or regional patient populations. The sites cannot provide the intimacy and personalization in health matters that naturally define the connectivity between patients and their local physicians. They cannot integrate telephone and direct access to the physician that are an integral part of the doctor/patient relationship. Privacy concerns weigh against sharing personal information with large impersonal Web sites. Moreover, teleconsultation, second opinions, and testing reports from any global location raise serious issues about reliability, reimbursement, and accountability.

To counter this development, local physicians have direct access to confidential patient information that can be posted on a secure channel or Web site connected directly to the patient. Modern information technology has offered medical group practices the capability to craft Web sites tailored to serve their own unique patient populations. National Web sites cannot easily duplicate this customization, which is supported by the trust and confidence the patient has in a personal physician.

The electronic age offers endless opportunities for open connectivity between a medical practice and the patient base it serves. As intranets and extranets evolve, most large medical groups will develop and maintain a secure virtual private network (VPN) to provide information resources and an interactive connectivity with their patients.

The e-commerce example serves to illustrate a powerful tool for physicians to commandeer a larger share of patients' total health care experiences and needs. Beyond prescriptive care, patients need access to information about disease entities and treatment options to make informed decisions. Most patients want to know as much as possible about their doctors and their practices. They are interested in physician credentials, convenience, expected outcomes, range of services, and so on. Patients want easy 24-hour access, privacy, personalized offerings, and the channels to voice complaints and be recognized. Most patients have a voracious appetite for information about lifestyle issues that promote wellness. A Web site efficiently provides all of this information. Modern Internet technology is a tool that assists the physician in proactively managing the patient relationship.

Most medical practices have computer hardware and software that support billing and, to a lesser extent, scheduling applications. To manage a wider range of activities (information sharing, decision making, proactive intervention, and continuity of care) requires an electronic system that provides a high degree of information capture, storage, and control. Without an effective information system, this is virtually impossible. The medical office that relies solely on a paper chart that must be created, filed, and individually retrieved and on verbal and handwritten transmission of information for practice interactions is poorly equipped to meet the challenges of managing the patient's entire medical experience. Electronic automation of the majority of processes is vital.

An adequate information technology infrastructure and platform is essential. The system should be designed to permit open connectivity between all the players. This includes front and back office, doctors, patients, hospitals, insurance companies, testing facilities, and so on. These conduits for open information exchange, interaction, and coordination are critical for a program that manages the patient relationship. Electronic technology is not the principal focus of this book, but we need to review some state-of-the-art requirements for an adequate information system:

✦ Ability to create and maintain a patient database that includes demographics, accounting data, diagnostic and procedural codes, e-mail addresses, and patient health risk profiles. In a typical office, the system would consist of a file server and a computer network. If the practice contracted with an application service provider (ASP) for software and Web services, desktop computers, file servers, and legacy systems could be replaced with network computers, wireless handheld devices, or other thin clients.

✦ Immediate direct and remote electronic access to pertinent patient information by authorized personnel and physicians via a local-area network (LAN) or wide-area network (WAN) configured as a virtual private network (VPN). Without Internet channels, this may be accomplished by using standard phone lines with software that connects computer to computer.

✦ Electronic capability to generate e-mail, fax, and patient notes to efficiently communicate laboratory and test results; inform about scheduled procedures and appointments; and generate follow-up reminders, patient instructions, prescriptions, and letters.

✦ A secure Web site that interfaces with the patient to provide and share information, answer questions, solicit complaints and feedback, offer additional services, and assist with case management.

- Fault-tolerant system that securely maintains and backs up patient files.

- If Web enabled, potential to comply with the Health Insurance Portability and Accountability Act of 1996 (HIPAA), the rules from which were finalized and took effect April 14, 2001, with a compliance date for physician providers of April 14, 2003. These include:
  - Provider and payer organizations must maintain access logs that show who is accessing data.
  - Health information, when transmitted via the Internet, must be encrypted, and the identities of the sender and the receiver must be authenticated.
  - Authorized persons must access computerized information using individual user names and passwords.

Some of the required features warrant further detail and definition.

An intranet is a window-based network that privately connects all personal computers in the practice. Using a browser or a direct connection link, the intranet can be ramped to the Internet via an Internet service provider (ISP). This supports e-mail and other services and provides the capability to maintain a Web site for publishing and hyperlinks that connect to other Web sites. Attractive Web sites are easily created. In a simple form, Web sites can serve to market the practice and to disseminate practice information through published brochureware.

An extranet is a secure Web channel between the medical practice or an intranet and outside partners. It can provide remote access for physicians and patients to confidential medical information. It also affords the capability to submit questions, give feedback, teleconference, document eligibility, schedule appointments, and receive answers. An extranet, like a commercial e-commerce site, can be used to purchase medical items or services. The capability for "cybervisits" and "telemedicine," in which a patient is monitored and treated via the Internet in the home setting, is evolving. With the advent of broadband transmission and multimedia capabilities, the possibilities of such a virtual private network are infinite. In the future, this may become one of the principal ways in which medical practices interact with patients. A logical long-term goal for a medical practice's e-commerce solutions is to facilitate a "one-stop shopping" destination for the patient that encompasses information resources, interaction, and service transactions.

E-mail, a means of fast, cost-effective, convenient two-directional communication on the Internet, offers a wide range of opportunities. As higher percentages of the population become Web-enabled, reminders, notices, and customized medical information can be sent by the practice electronically at virtually no cost and at a convenient time for the staff. The savings in time and effort in bypassing the telephone are considerable.

Fax and voice mail are an alternative to e-mail that also circumvent the conventional telephone call and do not require the use of the computer by the patient.

Electronic medical record (EMR) or computerized patient record (CPR): technology presents an opportunity for medical practices to achieve a paperless office while still fulfilling the needs for confidentiality, security, and back up.

The primary hurdle for physicians to accept EMRs is that electronically formatted documentation takes time. For physicians who may be accustomed to handwriting or dictating notes in abbreviated terms and who do not type, the demands may be burdensome. To facilitate data entry into an EMR, touch-screen and continuous voice recognition technologies are rapidly evolving. For the physician who wishes to dictate notes, portable electronic dictating devices can be used with later transcription, or, if devices are voice activated, notes can be downloaded into the medical record by a "correctionist." Memorized transactions and standard templates are widely used to speed the data entry process.

Remote access to the EMR by authorized persons is a distinguishing feature in advanced systems. The physician no longer has the encumbrance of scribbling notes for later entry into the chart and of carrying a notebook full of reminders. New handheld devices that are wireless and Web-enabled will further streamline the documentation process.

The applications within EMR programs can be introduced incrementally into a medical practice, with gradual integration and interfacing with other software applications. The electronic office system can be interfaced with other electronic networks to connect with a range of strategic partners via direct connection on the Internet. It is important that the partners have compatible systems that use standardized protocols.

Typical features of EMR programs include:

- ✦ Patient encounter information, including chief complaint, present illness, past medical history, family history, social history, review of systems, allergies, medications, physical examination, treatment plan, and instructions, can be entered. The sequence conforms to the standard process of the history and physical. A photograph of the patient can be scanned into the electronic chart to assist the staff in recognizing patients on arrival and in addressing them by name. The physician or a physician extender can enter the data by a handheld device, network computer in a treatment room, or at a central workstation. In some EMRs, a SOAP (Subjective, Objective, Assessment, Plan) format is used, and problem lists are created. The EMR can generate a comprehensive, legible medical record. A hardcopy day sheet to add to a paper record and patient instructions for the visit can be printed. Historical data, including allergies, medications, family and social history, and past diagnoses, can be easily updated and pulled from previous encounters.

- ✦ Many EMRs contain a coding application that records the number of bullets or data entry points to justify billed relative value units. This useful feature ensures appropriate coding and helps to protect a practitioner if subjected to a "fraud and abuse" audit by CMS.

- ✦ EMRs frequently provide a program to print prescriptions and fax or e-mail prescriptions to the pharmacy. Software applications for pharmaceutical control include flags that identify adverse drug interactions, lists that give correct dosages, and displays that exhibit the individual formularies for various MCOs.

- ✦ Most EMRs provide the capability to print customized patient instructions from memorized transactions and medical record entries.

- ✦ The option to create queues or lists of filtered phone calls by front office personnel targeted for specific physicians or employees is a frequent application that helps to ensure efficient call back and to avoid losing calls.

- ✦ Many EMR programs incorporate a scanning feature that uses electronic scanners, digital cameras, and digital movies to permit x-rays, graphics, and testing results to be scanned directly into the medical record. Optical character recognition (OCR) software permits data storage as text documents and avoids the problem of data reentry. A scanning capability is an essential application if the medical practice wishes to move to a paperless office.

- Most EMR packages interface with electronic billing and scheduling programs. This circumvents the need for double entry of patient information. Patients who fail to make or keep appointments can be identified and reminders can be electronically generated. The professional back-office staff can directly access the charge data.

- Graphs and charts of sequential critical lab values or physical findings to monitor patient progress and individualize treatment can be printed.

- EMRs become the repositories of large databases of patient information from which standard and custom reports containing up to 15 or more search parameters, including age, sex, ICD 9 and CPT codes, referring and treating physician, medication, allergies, physical findings, and so on, can be generated. This makes the EMR a data resource for clinical research, quality improvement, cost analysis, and tracking of a large range of variables.

- EMRs usually include a health maintenance application that tracks immunizations, routine screening tests, and preventive health care measures for individual patients. Basically, a health maintenance program provides tools to promote wellness and track continuity of care. In the process, patient connectivity with the medical practice is encouraged for provision of all health care services. Many programs have the capability to risk-profile patients on the basis of past medical and family history. This aids the medical practice in tailoring optimal lifestyle modification initiatives and screening for individual patients. A system of automated reminders and information sharing is developed that fosters continuity of care and tracks compliance. When properly implemented, a health maintenance program can micromanage a case management program for each patient (see Appendix B).

Many physicians may challenge the benefits of getting "wired" in their offices. To counter this, a quote from Microsoft Chairman Bill Gates is appropriate: "It will take a commitment by health care providers to reshape health care through digital information. The technology is available today," he says in his book *Business @ the Speed of Thought: Succeeding in the Digital Economy*. "An investment in a common infrastructure and tools will enable not just a huge reduction in costs, but better health treatment for everyone."

The Return on Investment from an Electronic Office

Conversion to a "wired office" with an electronic medical record and management system is a major undertaking. To put together the computers, storage devices, software, and communication network components of information technology requires significant investment in time and financial resources. Some monetary returns on investment can be directly measured, but the preponderance of benefits to the practice, such as streamlining of processes and information sharing, is difficult to quantify precisely in dollar terms.

Conversion effectiveness and functionality of the new system hinge on many cultural and structural factors in the practice. These include the commitment and involvement of the partners, expertise of the project team and quality of the information technology staff, expectations of the users, amount of organizational change required, and the threat to personal and vested interests. Implementation success also relates to the range of applications, user friendliness of the system, and the degree of alteration in patient flow and office processes.

In general, the cost savings that accrue from transactional changes within a practice are more easily identified than are returns from new strategic, decision support, and information sharing activities.

- Infrastructure to support the system usually consists of a client and server architecture and a network that links computers. An intranet can be created on the basis of the same technical standards as the Internet, and an extranet to interface with outside strategic partners can be developed to provide remote access. This produces a virtual private network (VPN) for the practice. The office network connection to the Internet supports Web publication and hyperlinks to other sites, e-mail, and surfing the Internet. Although direct financial return from building IT infrastructure is impossible to calculate, it supports activities that are measurable. Most important, a sound infrastructure offers a range of future options and the flexibility to exploit future opportunities.

- The standard features of an accounting and billing package introduce efficiencies of automated electronic billing and financial tracking. The number of staff hours saved is directly traceable.

- Other software applications with returns that are directly traceable and quantifiable include:

- Coding software ensures accurate coding. In most practices, this results in the submission of higher median codes to insurance companies for reimbursement.

- Data are directly entered into the electronic medical record. This eliminates or decreases transcription costs and standardizes the format for data entry. The latter aids in accessing and analyzing data.

- Electronic bulk purchasing and inventory control decrease purchasing expense and minimize inventories.

- Easy access to electronic patient information streamlines the search for patient data. It overcomes the delays inherent in office searches for paper charts. In a typical office, the chart to be pulled is either out of the file or misfiled 20 percent of the time. It often must be retrieved from stacks of charts awaiting addition of lab reports or other entries, review and physician signature, response to correspondence, and arrival of the day's patients. Moreover, remote connectivity enables information about patients to be shared between office locations. The transaction cost savings from eliminating these repetitive, non-value-added activities that often interrupt normal flow processes are measurable. In a typical office, it equals the time and efforts of at least one full-time employee (FTE).

- The "paperless" office eliminates the paper chart that must be created, filed, pulled, added to, and refiled. It minimizes the space necessary for paper storage.

- An integrated information system eliminates time-consuming, error-prone, and redundant data entry and documentation.

- The system can automate referrals, verify eligibility, generate and send prescriptions, manage testing results, and maintain call back and patient lists. Each of these features reduces the time spent on the telephone and in generating paperwork.

✦ Some returns are not easily measured. These include:

- Enhanced information sharing and patient education.

- Generation of a legible and organized comprehensive record that serves as a better legal document to defend against malpractice.

- Improved collaboration between partners and staff.

- Pathway to share information with other medical providers and partners.

- A formatted framework with which to introduce algorithms and critical pathways of care to better standardize and measure quality of care.

- Searchable databases that flag adverse drug interactions and drug recalls.

- Remote physician and staff access to patient and practice information.

- Data resources that assist in practice strategy and decision making.

- Information storage and management that supports the program to manage the patient relationship.

- Warehousing of charge data that permits cost analysis and projections to undertake profitable direct contracting.

✦ Last, information technology can be transformational for a medical practice. It can redesign the process and flow of the way in which work gets done, provide training resources, and support a "learning organization."

The financial rewards for a medical practice from electronic conversion and automation are compelling. The science of medicine is high-tech, and yet most medical practices operate as low-tech enterprises. Information technology exists today to fix the problem. Moreover, as newer technology becomes more user-friendly and less expensive, the conversion will become even more attractive. If medical practices seek to become capable management and information businesses, electronics holds the key. (See Appendix C for a Breakdown of the Dollars and Cents of an EMR.)

Implementing the Electronic Conversion

A critical mass of both professional and administrative personnel should be actively involved in planning and researching the IT project as well as the purchasing decision. Consensus among all associates to convert to an electronic office is essential. Once the decision is made to move forward, no hedging or back-pedaling is permitted. An installation and implementation plan should be crafted with a schedule for step-wise introduction that affords adequate training. All modification of office processes and changes in patient flow should be identified and solutions worked out before implementation. The scope and functionality of the program that is introduced should be well understood.

A number of issues need review when considering the purchase and adoption of a new electronic information system for a medical practice.

- ✦ Researching vendors on the Web is easily accomplished. Searches of medical software, electronic medical record, and applications service providers (ASP) will produce hundreds of sites. Prices are generally not listed. Most companies offer a free trial period and demonstration materials. Most of them provide a list of clients and contact references. Few offer a package that fully automates all aspects of the medical record. Integration with other applications and with the Internet are variable.

- ✦ There is a learning curve. It may take several months for physicians and staff to achieve mastery and smoothly navigate all of the applications. The implementation plan usually introduces the programs in a staged fashion.

- ✦ Computer and software vendors are prone to be overly optimistic about the capabilities of their products. They often promise unrealistic timelines and downplay the complexity attendant to implementation of the system. Consult with others who have used the system.

- ✦ Glitches, bugs, and crashes, along with networking and interface problems, are common during the first six weeks. Short vendor response times and timely support are extremely important during this period.

- ✦ Electronic medical record keeping places an increased burden of documentation on the physician. It requires time and tenacity to achieve the proficiency that maintains productivity. Regardless of the claims by EMR software vendors that the EMR permits a physician to see more patients per unit time, data entry usually consumes an additional minute or two of physician's time for each patient encounter. In a structured or template EMR, there are several mouse clicks, pen points, or verbal commands per encounter. Some or even most data entry can be delegated to the professional staff, transcriptionists, and "correctionists" to better distribute the workload.

- Many features of an EMR are immediate hits with the office staff. Because the EMR usually streamlines their work processes, their buy-in to the system's applications usually progresses smoothly. Unlike with the paper chart, multiple users can work on a medical record simultaneously.

- Front-end licensing fees and site costs for software from different vendors varies considerably. The package should be carefully costed by breaking it down into its component parts. Make certain all expenses are spelled out in the contract with the vendor. Research upgrade fees and support expenses and ensure that there is adequate provision for training.

- During the period of installation and implementation, an on-site temporary employee with complete familiarity with the system can decrease downtime, provide additional training, trouble-shoot problems, and minimize employee frustration. This proficient "techie" can be pivotal in ensuring a smooth transition to an electronic office.

- A thorough cost analysis should be a routine step when a practice is planning to purchase an electronic system. The up-front investment in the system is substantial, but the subsequent fixed, variable, and marginal costs are minimal. In most practices, capture of the initial investment costs is achieved within a year.

- As part of the process, the medical group must research the information technology capabilities of its strategic and trading partners to ensure that the new system can interface and network with their systems.

Computer skill levels in each medical practice vary widely and remedial training needs should be identified. In the ideal situation, the office manager, the managing physician partner, or the project champion is an avid computer buff and enjoys working out computer solutions. The implementation is facilitated if someone is appointed the "technology czar" or, more commonly, the chief information officer (CIO). This person "owns" the project and is assigned the duty to monitor installation and coordinate implementation.

The vast majority of information system investments that fail to deliver do so because they are poorly linked to organizational plans and goals. Information technology offers the tools but must be managed for a positive return. In constructing the "house of technology," if the objectives are poorly understood, the design flawed, and the carpenter unskilled; the quality of the hammer and saw are irrelevant.

Profitable Patients

To build the IT infrastructure and human resource capital to support a program to manage the patient relationship requires a substantial investment in time, effort, and money. Many of the internal processes of the practice require revision. New processes may alter patient flow and processing of patient transactions and interactions. To justify the expenditure, we need to examine the potential return on investment. This is critically important, because physicians are running a business.

In this light we need to identify the practice's most profitable patients in terms of lifetime value to a practice and whose improved health status increases physicians' professional satisfaction. How do we stratify patients who are most likely to connect with the program and provide a positive return on investment? How do we measure success, and what are the financial rewards?

Many barriers exist in the current medical marketplace that inhibit the health partnership between patient and doctor. Third-party payers may evaluate medical practices using token quality parameters to satisfy National Committee for Quality Assurance (NCQA) accreditation standards that suggest an emphasis on preventive medicine, but, in reality, MCOs restrict or disallow physician compensation for most preventive health care. Often, routine physical exams and wellness visits are uncovered services. Activities that constitute the art of medicine, such as empathetic counseling, holistic emotional support, and patient education, are uncompensated. Mental health services are minimalized. Financial incentives are heavily weighted toward interventional treatment and not predictive, preventive, and supportive care.

To understand the core problem, we need only appreciate that third-party payers' main focus is on the bottom line. Satisfactory financials hinge on minimizing provider reimbursements, restricting the range of care and coverage, skimming low-risk patients without chronic illness, and achieving successful price competition to capture the greatest number of enrollees. This intrusive macro-management of price incentives produces a profound market failure when we consider what patients need and value.

In 1997, one sixth of all eligible patients switched MCO insurance coverage. This produces a high level of physician switching that complicates a program to manage health care maintenance. Further compounding the problem is job mobility, patient geographic migration, medical insurers' mergers and acquisitions, arbitrary changes in a health plan's panel of providers, scarcity of health care dollars, and the uninsured, who often use the system only for urgent care. This churning of patient populations is debilitating for activities that manage a long-term patient relationship.

Disregarding these marketplace forces, can medical practices identify and target for their health promotion initiatives a segment of profitable patients whose loyalty generates a complete lifecycle of benefits for the practice plus the efficiencies of long-term care for established patients? In short, yes. The segmentation process is analogous to that in any business. To use search criteria for profitable clients in medicine may seem contrary to the societal mission of a medical practitioner. However, in the context of proactively managing an on-going relationship, it makes sense to focus a practice's resources on patients who benefit the most and who solidly connect with the practice. What criteria might be used to focus a medical practice on individuals who are more receptive to a long-term managed relationship?

+ Older patient populations that, when studied, have been found to be more loyal to their physicians, are more concerned about health matters, and have greater medical care needs.

+ Patients with compelling needs for medical supervision because of chronic conditions such as asthma, diabetes, or hypertension or histories of heart trouble, stroke, or cancer.

+ Patients with stable employment.

+ Patients who have lived in one community for many years.

+ Patients who express a strong commitment to pursue a healthy lifestyle.

+ Established patients who would switch their insurance coverage rather than switch physicians.

+ Patients who express a strong preference for the primary hospital to which the physician admits patients.

- ✦ Pediatric patients from conscientious families.
- ✦ Female patients who plan to enlarge their families.

What segments of patient populations might be less suitable for the program to manage the relationship?

- ✦ Patients who refuse to see the doctor except for urgent or emergency care.
- ✦ Patients who repeatedly miss appointments and/or do not accept advice or treatment.
- ✦ Patients who frequently switch physicians and health care plans.
- ✦ Patients who shop for their physicians and consider medical care a commodity.
- ✦ The difficult, narcissistic patient.
- ✦ The litigious patient.

These are very general classifications, but the concept of building a practice around stable patient populations to enhance profitability is valid. Only then can a long-term measurable return on investment (ROI) be achieved with health maintenance initiatives.

A practice's transaction costs to manage long-term established patients are much lower than those with new patients. Less new data entry is required either into the EMR or a paper chart. The office staff is familiar with the patient and can schedule more efficiently. The patient knows the policies, procedures, and processes of the medical practice. Fewer routine questions need to be answered. The physician knows the problem list, has a better intuitive grasp of the patient's behavior and medical needs, and can more effectively manage the patient. Historic information is easily accessible and does not have to be regenerated. Moreover, the physician is rewarded by the close personal relationship that develops with the patient over time.

To these mostly transaction cost savings, add revenues from:

- ✦ Regular wellness visits.
- ✦ Timely screening tests.

- Fewer missed appointments.
- Increased referral of friends and family members.

Plus, consider the intangible benefits that supporting the patient's entire health care experience gives:

- Cost containment provided by increased supervision of the patient's use of medical resources.
- The medical practice positioned as the exclusive source for patient information that empowers the patient to make better informed decisions.
- Guidance of the patient away from unproven therapies, marginal practitioners, and inappropriate medical care.
- Minimization of patient shopping for medical care.
- Control of referrals.
- Psychological rewards for the physician.

The concept of managing the patient relationship and forming a partnership in health care requires a genuine commitment from the patient. Once achieved, it provides a new definition of managed care in which the physician assumes the role of proactive manager. The patient is the beneficiary, and the relationship empowers the patient as controller of health care.

A medical practice can market a well-designed program as a patient privilege. Patients should be informed of the unique features and selection criteria for participation. Our new concept consolidates and coordinates comprehensive care under the auspices and direction of one exemplary medical practice that is rewarded by increased profitability and effectiveness.

Physician Stewardship: The Paradigm Shift

We've described "patient-focused strategies" for medical practices. The resultant service benefits directly accrue to the patient, from whom little is requested in return. The response from the patient is almost always positive. The patient effortlessly receives the benefits; whereas the medical practice receives the prescription to provide satisfying service.

In proactive management of the patient relationship to nurture a patient's life cycle functionality, a medical practice writes a prescription for change. The medical practice is the facilitator of change but the wellness prescription is given to the patient, who must make choices. The advantages accrue to patients if and when they adopt positive steps to responsibly direct their own health care.

To illustrate, let's look at the patient smoker. All individuals are bombarded daily with information about the hazards of cigarette smoking. They are keenly aware of the addicting properties, and most smokers have attempted to quit regularly. The physician who encourages the patient to stop smoking and offers to assist in the effort to quit is promoting behavioral change. The benefits for the patient result only if they actively change behavior. It is the patient's informed decision and choice. The practicing physician has the delicate balancing role of being supportive but nonjudgmental.

In urology practice, the author routinely gave smokers a hard sell about the benefits of smoking cessation. The arguments included capture of additional years of life and savings on the purchase of cigarettes. Perhaps 10 percent of patients were motivated to quit. Most patients who had no medical problems linked to smoking continued their habit. On the other hand when the patient had a bladder cancer that was directly attributable to cigarette smoking, the success rate rose to about 80%. This shows the willingness of patients to react to bad news with positive behavioral steps, but a reluctance to proactively quit prior to adverse consequences. We can extrapolate these observations to virtually all of the healthy lifestyle initiatives taken in managing the patient relationship. Some physicians may question why they should have to manage patients who resist changes in lifestyle. Nevertheless, if appropriate counsel and positive reinforcement can increase the percentage of patients who change their risky behaviors; the physician has fulfilled his or her duty and should feel justly gratified when a patient gives up unhealthy habits.

Although lifestyle counseling may seem meddlesome to the patient, it provides obvious value. The patient ultimately drives the change in behavior and makes choices; the physician and staff are only cheerleaders. Realistically, it is more difficult to motivate patients in preventive medical issues than to achieve compliance with medical treatment for illness.

This discrepancy between patient treatment and prevention responses often dampens the physician's enthusiasm for counseling on lifestyle issues. Moreover, positive results from lifestyle modification are derived in the long term and are difficult to quantify and measure. But the trust and intimacy of the doctor-patient relationship position the physician to be the most effective change agent in health matters. Health counseling should be considered an investment in the future, one that accrues returns over the patient's lifetime. Marketing healthy lifestyles is a difficult sell for the physician, but, when viewed through the eyes of the patient, yield long-term dividends that are equal to good prescriptive treatment.

Patients are independent contractors. They can choose to follow or not to follow advice and can make intelligent or foolish decisions. Physicians' role in health promotion is changed from their traditional role. Descriptors such as advisor, coach, partner, agent for change, and patient advocate aptly define this new role. The patient is the player.

This new paradigm gives the choice to the empowered patient. The patient is the decision maker. This may seem to mitigate the influence of physicians and take them outside the comfort zone of tangible results. In reality, patients are the best controllers of their health care and physicians must employ creative approaches to best support their health needs. Physicians have the resources to help patients make informed decisions. Their toolbox contains the behavior modification techniques of information sharing, reinforcement, encouragement, empathy, and repetition. Results are typically incremental, with inconsistent progress. The effects are not easily tracked, and the physician's desire for tangible quick results is often not met. However, this paradigm shift forms the basis for the best definition of patient-managed care and the "art of medicine."

Physician Time Constraints and Reimbursements

Two basic obstacles inhibit effective health promotion: physician time constraints and reimbursement.

Most health care plans provide little reimbursement for counseling and patient education. The ICD-9, CPT, and HCPCS billing codes for preventive medical services are convoluted and complex and charges are often not allowed. Screening and laboratory tests are most likely to be reimbursed, physical exams less reliably, and counseling least of all. All physicians, health care professionals, and consumers of health care must become lobbyists for systemic change that embraces compensation for and recognizes the value of preventive and predictive care. If resolved, this public policy issue will refocus the health care system on optimal health and lifetime functionality of the American public. On the demand side, patients make the choices, and educated patients are the best managers of their personal health. Health care policy should be the enabler and facilitator of transferring greater control to the patient. Payments to physicians for medical counseling, education, and relationship management support self-management that empowers patients to make the best choices.

With the vast assortment of demands on the physician's time and effort, any program to manage the patient relationship must automate and delegate as many routine interactions and activities as possible. This is a requirement if physician efficiency and productivity are to be maintained or increased. Physician extenders, including nurse practitioners, medical assistants, receptionists, and job-trained professionals, should be used extensively to actively support a wide range of services. The items that lend themselves to delegation will vary, depending on the type of practice and the orientation of physicians.

In reviewing a large number of medical practices, the author has always been surprised at how infrequently talented employees are empowered to actively provide repetitive, straightforward medical services. This is true even though the foremost tactic for a physician to increase productivity is to train "extenders" well, define the boundaries, and, whenever possible, delegate, delegate, and delegate.

The Patient Management Program

To some extent, traditional medical practices have always been service organizations that manage the patient relationship and provide resources for patient education and informed decision making. The traditional doctor/patient relationship encourages compliance and continuity of care. These activities are routine requirements to support prescriptive medical care.

In proactive management of the patient relationship, this existing relationship is leveraged to include ways to more closely monitor the patient's health and lifestyle, provide resources for patient education and instruction, and promote an interactive platform that strives to meet a larger share of the patient's health care needs. With the new approach, a medical practice could be viewed as the exclusive medical supermarket positioned to offer a wide range of services and support as well as treatment for the health care consumer.

Any program of patient relationship management must be creatively tailored for each practice's unique patient population. One size will not fit all. For instance, it is doubtful that lower socioeconomic or poorly educated populations will be connected to the Web or have fax machines. A medical practice would have to rely on printed materials and phone communication.

Four main categories of activity support a program that manages the patient relationship through information sharing and open connectivity.

✦ Patient education and providing medical information resources.

✦ Processes that support continuity of care.

✦ Improved connectivity and access to the physician.

✦ Interactive feedback and timely problem resolution.

Patient Education and Providing Medical Information Resources:

Medical information is available from a plethora of sources. Patients are exposed to a deluge of TV advertisements and medical segments on nightly news programs. New medical breakthroughs, novel diets for weight reduction, cholesterol control, adverse medical sentinel events, risks, fraud and abuse in the system, and so on are widely communicated in a wide range of formats. Often, reporting in the medical press unrealistically increases patient expectations. Additionally, it generates patient demands for new, unproven, or marginal therapies. The press frequently offers negative commentary about "greedy doctors" and adverse consequences of medical treatments that can instill distrust of the medical practitioner and the system. The media bias puts a sensational spin on medical information to attract viewers. Fragmented commentaries rarely give a balanced perspective about medical issues.

The media hype places the medical practitioner on the defensive. To respond, physicians must put things in perspective with balanced information that clearly defines the validity and the utility of specific medical information. They must counterbalance the media pull on the patient. This becomes an opportunity for the medical practice to provide reliable information to the patient—information that builds trust and confidence in doctors. What channels does the physician have to achieve this goal and fill the media's reliability gap? How can a medical practice, in a cost-effective manner, maintain a flow of information that augments connectivity with the patient?

To address this issue, let's examine four categories of information resources that enable a medical practice to maintain an educational conduit and connectivity to their patient populations.

- General practice information

- General medical information centered on timely predictive and preventive medical issues.

- Disease specific information

- Information about complementary and alternative medicine (CAM).

General Practice Information

The more a patient knows about a doctor and his or her medical practice, the greater the confidence level with that practice. And positive testimonials from a well-informed patient about a medical practice are more accurate and convincing. Shared practice information is a facilitator of patient intimacy that links to practice reputation.

Some of the means to disseminate practice information include:

- An office brochure that serves to market the practice and to introduce patients to the practice's outstanding features, services, and physicians as well as the policies and procedures of the practice. This brochure can be published on a web page.

- Newsletters or Web postings to inform patients about events, such as the arrival of a new associate, achievements and awards received by associates, new office locations, and new or more convenient medical services.

- Publication of practice performance data, such as exemplary patient satisfaction scores and treatment outcomes.

- Bulletin boards and wall hangings in the waiting room that feature information about the practice and show photographs of the physicians with brief biographical sketches.

| *Independence Day*

- ✦ Radio, TV, or print advertising. Although more expensive and not viewed positively by medical colleagues, promotional budgeting is becoming more commonplace.

Patients enjoy talking about their doctors; accommodate their wants and provide them with more practice information to share with their network of friends.

General Medical Information—Predictive and Preventive

Sharing health promotion/disease prevention information conveys the message that the physician is a partner in maintaining a healthy lifestyle. It positively reinforces healthy behaviors.

Reliable methods to achieve this objective include:

- ✦ Web page hyperlinks to medical Web sites or to authored articles by associates of the medical practice. Hyperlinks to Web sites should be researched to ensure truthful, unbiased, and comprehensive content that is easily accessed. Physician review is critical, because it is estimated that 20,000 medical Web sites exist, the content of which is essentially unregulated.

- ✦ Brief mailed, faxed, or e-mailed quarterly newsletter sent from the practice to provide information about timely subjects in areas in which the practice excels.

- ✦ Printed reference materials, such as wellness books, that detail lifestyle issues and give guidelines for what to do for common conditions and when an emergency arises.

- ✦ Health videos viewed on the waiting room TV, plus journals and handouts for patient consumption.

- ✦ Printed lists of suggested reading materials, article reprints, and a pamphlet that describes the practice's health maintenance program.

Granted, these initiatives often entail a shotgun approach, but they can serve to further connect the patient with the medical practice.

Disease Specific Information

These resources afford the patient immediate access to more comprehensive information about specific disease entities for informed decision making. Treatment options can be shared, realistic assessment of outcomes discussed to guide patient expectations, timely advice interactively provided, and immediate concerns addressed.

Vehicles to accomplish this objective include:

- Develop a patient information call center that provides a telephone or e-mail hot line to a nurse practitioner or trained professional who can filter and evaluate urgent problems, offer advice for minor medical conditions, and direct patients to information resources and appropriate care settings. These potential "command posts" can serve large group practices by being integrated with other practice initiatives, such as health maintenance, decision support, physician access and referral, appointment scheduling, continuity of care, and so on. The call center can be electronically configured as a common gateway to a full range of e-services offered by the medical practice. Additionally, interactive voice response (IVF) phone technology lends itself to the call center setting. If open 24 hours a day, a call center can circumvent the need for an outside answering service and give the patient improved access at all hours.

- Maintain a list of seminars and conferences that patients may attend that focus on specific diseases, such as diabetes, asthma, and heart disease.

- Train selected staff members to counsel patients about common disorders. These presentations should be designed to add to and reinforce treatment plans and instructions received from the physician.

- Give patients brochures and reference materials that provide reliable information about their illnesses. These may be generated internally or be supplied by drug companies or medical vendors.

- Provide group counseling and support groups moderated by staff members.

- Generate tailored and standardized computerized patient instructions that cover the 10 diagnoses that afflict 80 percent of patients.

There are infinite possibilities for a group practice to manage a program that actively disseminates disease-specific information to educate patients and promote compliance with treatment. A well-crafted program better positions the patient to make informed choices and, in the long run, saves the physician time, because knowledgeable patients require fewer detailed explanations. Additionally, most of the repetitious activities of informing can and should be delegated to staff members who act in the capacity of "physician extenders." Once the program is implemented, a staff member can assume the responsibility of managing the various initiatives.

Information about Complementary and Alternative Medicine

Complementary and alternative care is a growing industry, with a $27 billion price tag recently reported. A visit to the local library or bookstore reveals a vast assortment of book titles offering hundreds, if not thousands, of unconventional therapies with fancy names that confound the boundaries of Western Medicine. These therapies come with an extraordinary range of claims to prevent and ameliorate virtually all ailments. Myriad laboratories and paraprofessional practitioners have emerged to support this growing segment of the market. The FDA has declined to regulate the herbal market, presumably because of the wide range of unstandardized formulations, the paucity of scientific data, and the assumed safety of most herbal medications that are labeled nutritional supplements.

Many physicians have become involved with holistic or alternative medical care centers that employ some of the more efficacious complementary regimens, such as hypnosis, acupuncture, biofeedback, acupressure, massage, herbal medications, spiritual healing, and emotional support.

Alternate therapies have generated a following because they meet patient wants and needs. The time has passed when Western medicine can categorically disregard complementary medicine.

To manage this part of the patient's health care experience, a medical practice needs to understand and provide information about alternate remedies. It should promote complementary medicine when competent physicians provide it appropriately. A practice should also supply reliable information to counteract any inflated claims made by alternate therapists and therapies.

A holistic approach to medical care produces value for the patient. With careful management of the patient relationship, it should become the exclusive domain of the practicing physician.

Processes That Support Continuity of Care

Successful preventive medicine, health maintenance, and lifestyle management require regular patient office visits. How often have you heard the statement, "When I go to the doctor, all he does is take my blood pressure, so why should I make the effort to go?" A perfunctory pat on the back does not equal a satisfactory wellness visit. A health maintenance care visit should be instructive, with positive reinforcement of healthy behaviors based on health risk profiling. Physicians are trained to treat medical illness and consciously or unconsciously often have the mindset, "If it isn't broken, don't fix it." If physicians wish to manage a larger portion of patients' health care needs, they must espouse a philosophy that places greater emphasis on continuous connectivity and preventive medicine. Counseling and educating patients must assume equal importance to prescriptive care.

What tactics can the physician employ to achieve higher patient return rates and ensure seamless continuity of care? Some useful processes to achieve this goal include:

✦ Ticklers or alerts in the electronic health maintenance program that flag laboratory and screening tests that need to be performed. Filters in the program can search patient lists for these items and interface with a program of reminders to automatically notify patients.

✦ Postcard, e-mail, or telephone reminders of upcoming appointments generated by the scheduling program. This decreases the number of no-shows.

✦ Telephone calls or e-mailed messages to patients to evaluate responses to treatment and at the same time remind patients of their follow-up appointments.

✦ Post-operative telephone calls to check on patient status and discuss follow up.

✦ A comprehensive health maintenance package that is communicated to all employees and is firmly embedded in the office culture. All members of the staff should be empowered to act as missionaries for the program.

✦ Proactive telephone calls to discharged hospital patients to make their follow-up appointments and inquire about their progress.

✦ Electronically generate patient identification cards or ID bracelets that contain salient information about the patient in the event that he or she is being treated in the emergency department or in a facility out of the area. A smart card containing a comprehensive portable patient record offers infinite possibilities to ensure seamless medical care.

- ✦ A call center that has access to patient information in the EMR on which to base recommendations for patient compliance and follow-up.
- ✦ Free services, such as blood pressure check, cholesterol and osteoporosis screening, and medication samples, that keep the patient connected to the practice.

The basic point in focusing on continuity of care is to prevent any patient from becoming "lost" to the practice because of process errors, omissions, and breakdowns in communication. Any action that produces a stream of connectivity with the patient helps to ensure continuity of care.

Improved Connectivity and Access to the Physician

It is always difficult to balance the limited time constraints of the physician with the patient's need to have access and free counsel. For this reason, the professional component of the office force should be trained to effectively respond to phone calls. An experienced office nurse or medical assistant who stays within broad guidelines established by the practice can handle most calls.

One commonly used tactic to respond to medical questions that saves physician time is to have the medical assistant ask questions of the caller to define the nature of call and then state that he or she will check with the doctor and return the call. This adds the physician's authority to the response. If only the physician can address the issue and he or she is tied up, the caller should be given a time to expect the call to be returned. The patient should be asked when and where he or she can be reached. Emergency calls should be immediately directed to the physician, and the remainder should be queued for later callback. The patient should always be reassured that the physician "can be reached" and that no phone calls fall through the cracks.

Measures to improve efficiency in affording access include:

- ✦ An electronic phone queue that is part of the scheduling or EMR software program eliminates written messages and permits the physician to see in tabular form what calls need to be made at a later time.
- ✦ Regular call answering slots should be scheduled during which time patients know they can reach the doctor.

- Physicians who are out of the office should carry pagers and cell phones for easy access by the office staff. With cellular digital phones and personal digital assistants, new flexibility in communication is evolving. These devices will become Web-enabled and provide the physician with real-time access to all patient information and electronic messages.

- A medical practice should carefully examine after-hours coverage to ensure equivalent response from colleagues who cover the practice. A 24-hour call center is one way to ensure improved response to health care needs.

Interactive Patient Feedback and Timely Problem Resolution

As was stressed in chapter I, patient evaluation of the service quality of a medical practice forms the basis for service improvement. A practice should encourage constructive feedback and take measures to promptly address complaints. Interactive Web sites and call centers can assist with these efforts.

Preventive medical programs have been beset by problems with evaluation and measurement. Most controlled studies fail to substantiate direct medical cost savings from the preventive measures instituted by health insurance plans. When we view how insurance plans go about mandating preventive care, this is easily understood. To launch the plan, MCOs usually hire a group of new managers and develop an action plan that centers on a few critical measures of health promotion, such as mammography, Pap smear, and immunization rates. To control and evaluate physicians, they add these parameters to the "physician report card." In most instances, the program driver is fulfillment of NCQA accreditation requirements. Unfortunately, it adds a new layer of administrative expense with no change in reimbursement for the physician. Consequently, these programs are intrusive to the physician but ineffective in reorienting provision of preventive care. Patients' needs are not considered, and the essence of health promotion through counseling and education continue to be of subordinate importance.

For the physician, the many benefits of proactive management of the patient relationship are compelling. The goal of optimal health and life cycle functionality is synonymous with high-quality medical care. Practice financials improve with practice growth, increased revenues, increased referrals, good reputation, and the efficiencies of caring for informed patients. Of paramount importance, physician satisfaction and influence are enhanced.

The Information Asset

The greatest reward for medical practices from managing the patient's entire health care experience is often ignored. It is control of patient information. Information can be a group practice's most valuable asset. If large networked medical group practices are the primary repository of comprehensive patient information that accurately reflects the demand side of medical services and can organize these data, they know the composite picture of the customer. The essential patient information the author uses to analyze and forecast utilization behaviors is:

✦ Demographics, including age, sex, and occupation

✦ Current medications, including number and type

✦ Medical diagnoses

✦ Number of specialists seen yearly

✦ Major operations

✦ Number of minor operations

✦ Family history

✦ Social habits

Front-end patient information control is a powerful tool for physicians to craft strategies to influence the marketplace. This demand side information underlies success in direct contracting. Reflect on the possibilities. If you have access to the patient information listed above, could you build a formula that, within limits, predicts the patient's future consumption of medical resources? Could you reliably automate an information system to assign an economic risk for contracting to provide health care services for the patient? "Ownership" of confidential patient information affords medical groups a genuine competitive advantage that cannot be easily duplicated by other players.

Managed care organizations use historical charge data to "experience rate" employer groups. This retrospective data is used to set future health insurance premiums and assist the MCO in picking patient populations that consume fewer healthcare dollars. MCOs may use some basic demographic data such as age, sex, and occupation, in estimating their premiums. But forward-looking health care status and risk assessment of individual patients generally exceeds their information capabilities and is not factored in. Consequently, health insurance premiums often fluctuate widely year to year with quantum increases or decreases for employers at the termination of contracts.

In contrast to the MCO process, physician groups can potentially underwrite health coverage on a better-substantiated prospective basis. They possess more complete patient information that includes past medical, family, and social history from which to make projections. Likewise, on the provider supply side, they have comprehensive data about patterns of practice and resource consumption of their physicians. Medical practices can undertake a rating process analogous to an insurance actuary who forecasts risks on the basis of complete data. Each parameter of patient information could be assigned a weight. In the aggregate, a weighted average could be derived for contracting with enrollee populations. Information technology makes this an achievable goal.

Chapter 3

Control of Health Care Costs: A Physician's Prescription

"I have excellent medical insurance and keep abreast of the latest medical developments through the nightly news programs and alternative medicine Web sites. I frequently switch doctors because they do not order the tests I feel are necessary or refuse to refer me to specialists. I take 12 prescription medications from four doctors, have had six elective major surgical interventions, and have visited outside cancer screening, spine, and sports medicine clinics during the past six months. My group of specialists routinely screens and aggressively treats with the most advanced techniques." Can health care costs be managed in this type of patient?

MCOs, federal and state government, employers, and other agencies have attempted to contain medical costs using the macromanagement framework of managed care and competitive market forces. This has not achieved the desired results. Health care costs continue to rise and currently consume about 14 percent of the gross domestic product (GDP). Contrast this with 1950, when health care costs consumed 4.4 percent of GDP. In recent years, the annual increase in health care costs has exceeded the annual increase in the consumer price index (CPI) by one or two percentage points. National health expenditures in the year 2001 were projected at more than $1.3 trillion, with hospital care accounting for 33 percent and physician services 20 percent.

In spite of these expnditures, health care statistics for the United States do not outshine those of other developed countries whose expenditures consume less than 10 percent of their GDPs. What explains this discrepancy, and what measures can be considered to afford more value for money spent on the U.S. consumer of health care?

Federal health care programs and policy have fostered an "excess supply state" across all health care services. Resultant redundancies and unregulated excess capacity on the supply side have led to an explosion in demand for health care services. A plethora of providers fuel the demand through aggressive marketing and media exposure to the alleged medical benefits of new developments. The physician can prescribe from a cornucopia of medical options. With little understanding of the limitations of medical treatments, the consumer is easily seduced by a universe of great expectations.

Economic evaluation shows that most prescriptive medical care is price inelastic. Real health care needs are compelling and finite; cost is usually of secondary importance and does not alter demand. As an example, the diabetic needs insulin. It would be inappropriate and dangerous to postpone the purchase of insulin because of price. Additionally, health insurance removes price from most purchasing decisions.

Physician practice revenues approximate 13 percent of the total health care bill, and about half of these receipts are spent on office overhead. Yet physicians direct 80 to 85 percent of all health care expenditures through micro-management of medical care for individual patients. Consequently, this role in health care allocation gives the individual physician the ability and the ultimate responsibility to contain health care costs. It is the physician's evaluation that dictates resource utilization.

In the 1980s, many medical commentators conveyed the message that "whoever has the gold controls the system." This implied that third-party payers who controlled reimbursements and providers who were richly endowed had the power to dominate the medical system. Physicians who collectively had little "gold" were seemingly relegated to secondary player status. Is this assertion true? In the highly technical field of medicine, the physician possesses the intellectual capital. He is fundamentally unchallenged in prescribing appropriate care and in developing standards of medical care. Consequently, the physician in business terms is in charge of inputs and conversions in the system and also shoulders responsibility for outcomes. The physician may not have the "gold," but he or she has the authority. The physician is the player with the capability and the duty to contain costs in the medical system.

The market forces of price competition and managed care are not working to control costs beyond one-time savings captured by decreasing provider reimbursements and limiting the range of covered medical services. The medical marketplace, however, has been shown to be unyielding to conventional economic theory and macro-management, and this approach has produced and perpetuated mainly market failure. Managed care and price competition have had little positive impact on the practicing physician who micro-manages one patient at a time.

If the responsibility to contain costs falls to physicians, what strategies can be used to achieve cost efficiencies in the system and restrain costs? We need to review the causes for high resource utilization and waste and then craft physician solutions that eliminate unnecessary expenditures and contain costs.

Cost Awareness

In most instances, physicians have little understanding of what things cost, even though they keep fairly accurate records about rates of reimbursement and office expenses. The cost of medical care is rarely discussed between physicians and patients. Other than with medications, few instances occur in which a treatment decision is made on the basis of cost considerations. Only a handful of patients ask the the doctor what their care will cost. This indifference to cost is remarkable, because rising medical care costs have been the main driver of the transformation of American medicine during the past 20 years. The culture within medicine seems impervious and immunized to cost considerations.

Why is cost such a subordinate issue in medical practice, and what can be done to elevate the level of cost awareness? If physicians and patients knew what every test, admission, referral, and procedure they ordered cost, the mere awareness would lead to voluntary measures to squeeze waste out of the system and search for more cost-effective remedies.

✦ Physicians and patients with insurance perceive that they spend other peoples' money (OPM) in the consumption of health care services. In general, there are no penalties or financial disincentives for a physician to prescribe unduly high cost health care. Likewise, after employers pay the insurance premium, patients have no incentives to curtail the amount of health care they consume. To address this disconnect between cost and service, physicians and patients need to start viewing every dollar spent on health care as a scarce commodity coming from their own pocketbooks. To enhance cost awareness, we would suggest that, on every wage payment stub, employers list the dollar amount paid for health insurance and how this reduced the employee's wages. And there should be a process by which physicians are made aware of the total costs incurred in treatment decisions. These activities would bring cost into focus.

- In the medical school curriculum, there are few courses that focus on the costs of medical care. How can physicians be expected to contain costs when they have not been trained to know what the costs are? The importance of cost/benefit ratios in medical care must become a standardized part of the medical school curriculum and of residency training. Cost appreciation is not an inherent personality trait; it is a learned behavior.

- At medical conferences and seminars, medical society meetings, and scientific sessions, cost is rarely mentioned when papers are presented. It seems reasonable that all medical conferences devote some time to cost considerations and cost/benefit analysis. This would enhance the ability of physicians to factor in cost. Physicians must be able to identify and analyze what it costs before they can take steps to become more cost efficient.

Cost increases are the Achilles' heel of the medical profession, and the physician's indifference to cost is probably the most insidious—as well as the most remedial—driver of costs. To address this issue, we need to craft a model that uses dynamic economic data alongside clinical inputs in the development of treatments and recommendations. Physicians would respond decisively and appropriately to a "cost" message when presented in parallel with the other consequences of therapy.

First Dollar Coverage

After payment of the medical insurance premium, patients with no out-of-pocket or minimal point-of-service expense tend to place more demands on medical resources. This is exemplified by indemnity health insurance with first dollar coverage, which requires a higher premium than other forms of health insurance. Studies have shown that individuals with a significant coinsurance payment will spend up to 25 percent less than a beneficiary with first dollar coverage. It is human nature to place less value and utilization restraint on a service that is seemingly free.

Twenty percent of Americans consume 80 percent of health care dollars. Lacking financial restraints, many patients have enjoyed the luxury of seeking doctors' advice for trivial complaints, pushing for the most expensive and elaborate tests for minor ailments, and insisting on treatments that provide minimal benefits. Some patients have come to view the trip to see the doctor as a social occasion. This burden on the system raises health care costs for everyone.

Health insurance carriers use copayments, deductibles, and partial payment plans to address this problem in a limited fashion. A better solution is to have patients spend their own money. They make the choices, and health care consumers are the best managers of their own care. "Defined contribution" plans, in which employers provide a "benefit account" for employees to spend on their own health-care, is one logical approach. Medical savings accounts (MSAs), tax credits, and other plans that enable the patient to accumulate a reserve from which to pay for health care encourages prudent choices and serves to introduce real price competition into the medical marketplace. Individuals are prone to spend their own money wisely and can be a major enabler of a cost- efficient system of health care.

Aging Population

Statistics clearly show that the mean age of the population is increasing as the "baby boomers" reach middle age. Older individuals consume more medical resources. The number of inpatient hospital days is about three times higher in a Medicare population than with younger enrollees. There is no solution to this demographic reality, which will place an increasing burden on the system.

Several years ago the "Oregon Plan" was devised for Medicaid enrollees in that state. Health care services were rationed on the basis of prioritization of diagnosis-related groups (DRG) in order to contain health care costs. The plan acknowledged the scarcity of health care dollars in the state budget and offered coverage for 467 higher priority DRGs that fell within budgetary constraints. Recipients, if they wanted uncovered services, often migrated to other states. Inflexible and arbitrary features in the plan were controversial and in general poorly received by the public. Moreover, such a plan is subject to political manipulation in determining what services are necessary. Thus, for both young and old, explicit rationing of medical care does not seem to be an acceptable approach. Americans want choices and the freedom to make their health care decisions.

Health promotion programs to improve the general health status of the population would seem to be a more logical direction for health care policy. A healthier population would place fewer demands on the system and, in the short term, decrease health care costs. Theoretically, if you could postpone the age of onset of illness to closer to the age of death, you could compress morbidity into a shorter period, thereby decreasing medical expenses. However reasonable, it is uncertain that, in the long term, this would decrease overall medical spending on senior citizens.

Medical Technology

New technologies that breed medical interventions and screening tests plus new pharmaceuticals have a profound effect on medical care costs. A large range of vendors who produce these goods and services use elaborate push and pull marketing strategies to drive the new technologies. Remarkably, three of the eight companies with the largest national advertising budgets are pharmaceutical companies that, for the most part, market directly to the consumer through television ads. Patients are directly influenced through the media to request these new, often expensive, and sometimes unproven remedies.

Moreover, new technologies often become available and integrated into medical practice before careful cost-utility analysis is performed. National medical societies and physician organizations frequently compound the problem, because they traditionally view new technologies as a means to expand their scope of services, command a larger share of the research and health care dollar, and gain national exposure via the media. Physicians like the prestige and market visibility of being early adopters of new technology. Additionally, compensation for newly introduced procedural codes is generally higher than for established procedures.

Academic physicians have joined the patent game and formed partnerships with venture capitalists and even academic institutions to commercialize academic findings. Federal initiatives support these activities with taxpayers' dollars.

To counterbalance these marketing excesses and vested interests, a new control process for the introduction of new technology seems warranted. Entrepreneurial ventures should not be permitted to enter the medical environment without comprehensive review. It would seem appropriate for health care policy on the federal level to lead the way in the responsible introduction of new technology. Review boards that use information databases and committees of impartial experts should evaluate the costs and the utility to the consumer before unleashing new technology. Well-controlled clinical trials should be held to high standards of statistical validity and confidence, and independent investigators should be called upon to interpret the results and evaluate the benefits. To some degree, the National Institutes of Health (NIH), the Food and Drug Administration (FDA), and the Centers for Disease Control and Prevention (CDC) perform these functions, but their efforts are highly fragmented, often controversial, and frequently in conflict with vested interests. Moreover, NIH and other federal agencies that distribute federal research dollars support unregulated proliferation of medical technologies in the marketplace.

Some would argue that greater oversight and accountability would stifle innovation and investment in new technology. This argument has some validity, because the private sector invents and supports most of the new breakthroughs and basic research in medical science. In response, however, we could argue that a centralized federal initiative could be designed to facilitate scientific research without increasing burdensome paperwork and red tape. One centralized agency could coordinate the efforts and objectives of the many fragmented regulatory and financing health care entities. It could promote fair and appropriate distribution of federal research dollars, open access to the body of scientific information, encourage free exchange of information between investigators, and guarantee the efficacy and effectiveness of new technologies. It would better focus health care policy on benefits to the health care consumer.

In the current medical environment, implementation of new technology is fragmented and often haphazard. In many instances, marketing drives adoption rather than critical assessment and consensus. The nation's health is too important for this disconnect to continue.

The FDA mainly reviews human safety issues and treatment efficacy in defined populations under ideal circumstances in approving new technology and medications. Economic outcomes and cost-utility ratios are only peripherally examined. Effectiveness in typical populations under average circumstances is not considered, and comprehensive clinical guidelines are not crafted to assist the practicing physician. Moreover, once a new technology is approved for one application, it is often adapted to other applications without further critical review. It is obvious that any review process should look at all criteria, including costs, benefits, and quality of life issues, prior to certification for general use.

To illustrate, we will use one of the processes by which a new surgical procedure is introduced to medical practice. Collaborating with physician investigators, a vendor develops a new application for an existing surgical device. FDA approval is not required, because the medical device used in the hypothetical new procedure has previously been approved for other applications. The preliminary clinical study on a small group of patients results in publication of several articles in the medical literature. The results are also presented at medical society meetings to familiarize physicians with the new procedure. In the next phase, the principal investigator, with the financial support of the vendor, sponsors training seminars for interested physicians. The registration fees at these one- to three-day seminars are high, and they provide some, but limited, hands-on experience. A certificate of attendance is given to the physician registrant, who feels confident that he or she can capably perform the new procedure. Upon returning home, the physician asks the hospital to purchase new equipment to carry out the new procedure. Customarily, no budget, cost analysis, or quality assessment summary is submitted. Approval by the institutional review committee (IRC) is not required because the procedure is not investigational. The hospital administrator is expected to trust the physician's judgment and promise that the new technology will increase hospital utilization. The equipment is purchased. Other practicing physicians in the community hear about what their colleague is doing. They perceive a competitive disadvantage if they are not qualified to do the new procedure and attend the course. They spread the technology to their respective hospitals. Thus, the new technology becomes institutionalized across all hospitals. Often, no one stops to consider whether the new procedure produces real value for the patient. Moreover, there may be a steep learning curve to a new procedure with an insufficient caseload to ensure physician proficiency. This unstructured "trial and error" approach to introducing new technology often produces a high rate of morbid complications. Most patients prefer that their doctors not "practice" on them.

In the surgical field, new treatments often come and go, almost like fads. Over the past decade, 25 or more creative new medical and surgical treatments have been described and employed to treat benign enlargement of the prostate (BPH). There remains little solid data that supports one over the other, and most often the investigator's bias rules the day. There has been little general agreement as to cost effectiveness and outcomes. Consequently, any treatment meets the standards of care criterion.

These scenarios are typical. During most of the process, no attention is given to cost analysis, and rarely are cost-utility ratios thoroughly debated and critically reviewed. There is a need for new processes to establish standards that more uniformly ensure a satisfactory cost/benefit ratio.

On a more positive side, the author speculates that, at some future date, medical technology will begin to decrease health care costs. Newer electronic technology accounts for most of the increase in productivity enjoyed by our society. Perhaps future medical innovations will streamline diagnosis, afford cost-effective mass screening for disease, and decrease the cost per life year saved. The future will probably hold many pleasant surprises.

Unnecessary Surgeries and Other Medical Interventions

To determine what is necessary and what is unnecessary requires a complex judgment call for each medical treatment decision. The incentives in a fee-for-service and first-dollar coverage environment favor doing more rather than less. Moreover, patterns of practice vary widely. Risk-adjusted severity of illness indexing within patient populations also complicates comparisons among providers in utilization of medical resources.

Let's use the treatment of routine inguinal hernia as an example. Many millions of Americans have a groin rupture or hernia. Hernias can produce pain, increasing bulges, and even hospitalization requiring urgent or emergency surgical repair. However, most of them are asymptomatic and may or may not progress over time. Should the mere presence of a small inguinal bulge be sufficient indication for hernia repair that entails anesthesia, time from work, postoperative pain, a sizeable hospital bill, and minor risk? It is standard medical practice for surgeons to repair all detectable hernias. This example is representative of a wide range of gray areas in surgical interventions that incur significant expense with minimal benefits.

On the medical side, practitioners often treat minor elevations in cholesterol with no additional risk factors with expensive medications rather than counseling about dietary factors and exercise and prescribing less expensive remedies, such as Metamucil. The combined wholesale sales of Zocor and Lipitor, the two most commonly prescribed medications for cholesterol control, were $5.2 billion in 1999 or almost one half of one percent of all health care expenditures. Likewise, mild essential hypertension is often treated with antihypertensive medication without counseling about weight reduction, cigarette smoking, and dealing with daily stress factors. We need to ask what is more beneficial for the patient, expensive medication or lifestyle counseling?

Herbal medicines and lifestyle drugs raise additional issues with regard to therapy at the margin. Americans spend about $5 billion per year on herbals, at a rate that is increasing 18 percent per year. In Germany, more than half of all prescriptions are written for herbal medications. No hard data exist to support the use of herbal medications when viewed from the perspective of customary medical practice, standardization, and FDA approval. The need for greater safeguards for the public that consumes these unpredictable and often toxic remedies is obvious. The physician has a pivotal role in regulating their usage.

Cosmetic surgery (e.g., hair transplant, refractory eye surgery, tummy tuck, liposuction, spider vein ablation, and face-lift) raise additional issues about demand-driven utilization. It is virtually impossible to quantify the emotional benefits versus the cost and risk.

The fundamental problem with cosmetic surgery and herbal medications is that demand and consumption are driven by aggressive marketing, peer pressure, fads, media hype, narcissism, and compulsive behaviors—a Pandora's box when one critically reviews ways to contain costs. However, it should be noted that, with these therapies, the patients make the choices. Because it is usually an out-of-pocket expense, the consumer places a real monetary value on the service.

Overall, aggressive treatment of marginal conditions produces marginal value plus considerable expense. Philosophically, in the current medical environment, commission dominates omission. We need a new, balanced approach.

Some commentators report that 30-35 percent of surgical interventions are unnecessary or produce very limited benefits when viewed from the standpoint of patient risk, quality of life, and expense. Excepting a few high-volume standardized interventions such as C-section or coronary artery bypass surgery, the definitive indications for many surgical interventions are fuzzy and subject to the individual doctor's interpretation. The physician can easily mold the clinical picture to meet the mandatory prior authorization requirements of third-party payers.

Concurrent and retrospective case review conducted by quality review committees (QRC) and morbidity and mortality (M&M) conferences produce inconclusive data that rarely solve a utilization problem. Too often, these hospital committees focus solely on sentinel events, deaths, and risk management while not addressing significant variations in patterns of practice and resource consumption.

Medical directors and department heads are often impotent in addressing utilization problems. Reasons for this include situations in which the department director may be the main offender. Moreover, collegial behavior; threat of retaliation and legal action when sanctioning a colleague; the very nature of the thankless, stressful task of policing the department; restraint of trade issues; and time constraints are barriers to effective monitoring of peer behaviors. Without better defined standards of care, the problem is virtually unsolvable in the current hospital medical staff structure.

To put things in perspective, it is the individual physician's intellectual honesty and integrity that are the best guarantors of appropriate intervention. In the current environment, it is difficult to uproot and sanction the physician who is focused on financial gain and gaming the system.

On the optimistic side, peer pressure and statistical analysis of practice patterns can encourage cost-effective behaviors. As large medical practice groups form, with information systems that track practice data and afford the capability to generate standards, the mandate to control costs will cause unnecessary interventions to be increasingly scrutinized. The gaming physician will no longer be able to hide under the shield of ambiguity and poorly defined standards of care.

Oversupply of Medical Providers and Facilities

Nature abhors a vacuum. Excess capacity in medical services encourages excess utilization, or, stated differently, "supply drives demand." Most observers believe that, to limit the growth of expenditures in the health care system, measures to control the supply side of the equation are more effective than measures to control the demand side. Analysis of rising costs during recent years gives credence to this thesis.

The physician who directs patient care can "churn" and create clinical loads by increasing the number of office visits, tests, and interventions for each patient. Moreover, physicians who over-utilize have an increased number of patients with morbidity to manage.

Debates rage about whether or not there is an oversupply of physicians and about what the ratio of specialists to primary care physicians should be. Enabled by the federal government, in the past 30 years the output of physicians from our medical schools has increased well in advance of our increasing population. The apparent logic behind this federal mandate was that, by increasing the number of physicians, there would be improved distribution of doctors and increased price competition to drive down health care costs. Unfortunately, the medical marketplace did not adhere to this textbook competitive model and the opposite has occurred.

Moreover, the number of foreign medical school graduates practicing in the U.S. has been increasing. In 1997-98, 32.9 percent of all the resident physicians in Ohio were international medical school graduates (IMGs) compared to only 12.1 percent less than a decade earlier. In 2000, 10,703 of 25,056 physicians participating in the National Residency Matching Program were graduated from foreign medical schools.

Federal legislation, mainly the Hill-Burton Act of 1946, has caused the same excess supply scenario to develop with hospitals by dramatically increasing the number and dispersion of hospital beds. Additionally, hospitals have accumulated large "war chests" of retained earnings to add bricks and mortar to their systems and exploit market opportunities. This has further exacerbated the oversupply of hospital beds and services that add cost to the medical system. In some regions, hospital occupancy rates average 50 percent or less.

It is apparent that health care policy should include regional planning that limits this unbridled explosion in hospital services. Although of limited success in the past, a system of certificates of needs (CONs) and permits for expansion and services should be considered part of systemic planning. The defined role of hospitals in the marketplace should be inpatient "cost centers." Hospitals have historically been poor "organizers" of health care, and, in general, these "not-for-profit" institutions are focused on profit and are often not friendly to the patient-consumer.

The long-term solution to the oversupply of physicians is fairly simple. Decrease the throughput of physicians graduating from U.S. medical schools, limit the inflow of IMGs, eliminate marginal residency programs, and decrease the numbers of specialty residents. Study and substantiate the supply needs for physicians, callously ignore the political lobbyists, disregard fragmented conflicting data, and seek the optimal number of physicians. Continue to offer incentives to physicians to practice in underserved areas. The central goal should be to make each physician sufficiently busy that he or she is motivated to provide only services with an appropriate high cost-utility ratio and does not need to focus on ways to maintain income.

The problem with excess hospital bed capacity and services is more difficult to solve. Because payroll is the major expense for hospitals, most hospitals have staying power and the unique ability to decline profitably. When experiencing a declining census, the hospital simply cuts staffing. Decreasing hospital reimbursements can stress hospitals. This may drive hospital administrators to consider repositioning their institutions through mergers and acquisitions, but it is difficult to force these not-for-profit institutions to close their doors. The current hospital system is highly decentralized and fragmented; consolidation to achieve economies of scale and scope should be encouraged. Some have suggested that struggling hospitals be turned into prisons; this is not altogether a crazy idea.

The goal of health care policy should be to bring all of the marketplace players together on the same page to work collaboratively to solve excess supply problems. The medical environment needs to be less fragmented with more consensus building and systemic planning.

Medical Practice Overhead

Office expenses have been increasing moderately because of many factors, including inflation, higher equipment and supply costs, rising malpractice premiums, increasing burdens of paperwork, higher employee pay and skill levels, and the initial costs attendant to office automation.

In an environment of declining reimbursement for medical services, one of the first knee-jerk responses from physicians is to decrease office overhead in order to maintain income. This may be conventional fiscal logic, but it often produces profound negative effects on service, efficiency, and productivity. Decreasing employee pay, downsizing the office force, and arbitrarily expanding job responsibilities can lead to high employee turnover rates, low office morale, and decreased efficiency.

The salient issue is that strict containment of office expenses is often counterproductive. Hiring, training, and retention of loyal employees with the requisite intellectual and emotional capital are a cost-saving strategy. Too often, medical practices just look at the bottom line numbers, with little understanding of the staff loyalty effect that affects overall operations and customer service. A highly motivated office staff is a practice's greatest asset. Medical practices need to employ the best talent available—talent that conserves physician time and buffers the physician from the hassle factor by effective complaint resolution, smooth process perfection, and empowerment to assume the role of physician extender.

Moreover, medical practices should look to new information technology to increase office productivity. The efficiencies of streamlining office processes can decrease the number of employees needed without affecting operations.

Consolidation into larger group practices offers operational efficiencies and economies of scale. Office payroll expenses for larger group practices, as a percentage of revenues, run five to ten percent below those for smaller groups.

In general, the strict ratcheting down of office expenses is often penny-wise and pound-foolish. If anything, medical practices need to spend more on building an office infrastructure that efficiently conducts medical practice.

MCO Administrative Expense

MCO administrative, marketing, and underwriting expense and profits consume a whopping 20-25 percent of health care premium dollars. What does the medical system receive in return for this bureaucratic control? Very little, aside from systemic stress and feeble, superficial attempts at macro-managing the quality of medical care. When MCOs entered the marketplace, there was a need for an "organizer" of health care. However, through physician development of large medical group practices and technology infrastructure, MCOs are becoming vestiges of inefficiency, excess bureaucracy, market failure, and sunk costs. By eliminating the redundancies of the third-party system, adding the efficiencies of large group practices, and incorporating the productivity gains from information technology, administrative costs should not exceed five to ten percent. Elimination of 15 percent of health care costs is a significant savings.

Patient Expectations

Patients expect more from their doctors. This is a positive force when viewing a medical practice from a service perspective. However, the pull marketing strategies used by product manufacturers, pharmaceutical companies, hospitals, and ancillary providers to stimulate needs and enhance demand encourage inappropriate use of marginal therapies with little regard to cost and efficacy. The physician and informed patients provide the best barrier to this unacceptable use of medical resources. Physicians are patient advocates when they thwart patient efforts to seek exotic or unproven medical remedies.

The High Cost of Dying

CMS reports show that 28 percent of Medicare and Medicaid expenditures are for those over age 65 in the last year of life. This approximates 18 percent of lifetime costs for medical care. Pneumonia is no longer the "old man's friend and the young man's enemy." The tenor of the times is that all medical conditions should be treated aggressively, with limited regard to quality of life issues. G-tube placement, parenteral nutrition, amputation, relief of bowel obstruction, intubation, and ICU management are commonplace in treating the terminally ill who have no hope for any quality of life. Often, this aggressive treatment clouds the act of dying with unnecessary pain and suffering and prolongs the anguish for the family.

According to a *Time/CNN* poll, 7 of 10 patients wish to die at home, although three-quarters die in medical institutions. At least one third of patients spend 10 days in intensive care units during their final days. The warm home environment affords a more comforting demise than the sanitary hospital, where death occurs among strangers.

What are some of the causes that drive excessive aggressive care for the terminally ill?

- ✦ Physicians are trained to preserve life, and many of them have very conflicted feelings about death and dying. Rarely is a primary physician at the bedside when death occurs.

- Family emotions and conflicts always come into play when a close relative is dying, and sometimes guilt and grief are difficult to manage. In many instances, the family wants everything done and, in general, the more dysfunctional the family (usually families that have out of town siblings who have not seen their parent for months or years), the more is requested for a dying relative. With caring families, the decision to withhold treatment at the extremes of life is more easily made in consultation with the physician. Physician counseling becomes of critical value to ensure that only rational supportive treatment is carried out.

- Quality of care measures and rating systems for nursing homes and emergency departments (EDs) are pegged to mortality rates. Often in the nursing home setting, if terminally ill patients (demented, bedridden, incontinent, decubiti, and so on) develops pneumonia, sepsis, or urinary tract infection, they are promptly sent to the ED. If possible, no patient is permitted to die in the nursing home, because it will reflect unfavorably on the statistics. The same holds true for the ED, where comprehensive evaluation and treatment is routinely initiated on the terminally ill. If the patient arrests, a full code to resuscitate is performed. Once admitted to the hospital these patients are difficult to rehabilitate to a level where they are suitable for discharge back to the nursing home. The logistics of finding a nursing home that will accept them often take several extra days of hospitalization. Additionally, a hospital is a dangerous place, with hospital-acquired infection, medical mistakes, and falls frequently occurring in these confused and compromised high-risk patients.

   When aggressive treatment has no benefit other than prolonging a tormented existence by hours, days, or a few weeks, is this ethically good or does it do harm? Quality measures need to be crafted for nursing homes and emergency departments to permit death with dignity. A hospice approach to maintain patient comfort is reasonable, and the concept of supportive comfort and palliative care should be expanded to a wider range of medical service environments. Physicians must master this new pathway of care to eliminate waste and suffering in the dying process.

- Primary care physicians and specialists often do not like the frustration and emotional discord of caring for the terminally ill and individuals with incurable degenerative end-stage disease. They often refer these patients to other specialty providers, who, in turn, feel they must further evaluate and institute a new round of treatment. A recent survey found that three of five physicians treating dying patients had known the patient less than a week. Despite the diminishing returns, it is a very difficult decision to stop the rounds of referral and treatment and provide only supportive care. It should be the primary treating physician's duty to act as the filter that prevents unjustified treatment with no benefit.

✦ Once a patient is on life support or has had a surgical intervention, the physician feels obligated to continue aggressive treatment. In some 10 percent of patients, even advanced directives from a living will are not followed. Legal and moral safeguards make it difficult to terminate treatment without absolute proof that no potential benefit exists. Ethics committees and treating physicians should coordinate efforts to do what is appropriate and makes sense for the patient.

The main point is that, through contact, consultation, and consensus, patients should be permitted to die with dignity and comfort, and at home if possible in a way that does not waste medical resources. A close bond with a primary care physician is essential to achieve this goal. Quality of life should be the central concern.

Pharmaceuticals

Prescription drug prices are the most rapidly rising medical expense segment. During the 1990s, pharmaceutical costs rose from $38 billion to more than $110 billion today. Excessive drug company profits have stirred a lively controversy over pharmaceutical advertising budgets, patent expirations and extensions, R & D expense recovery, and generic medications. This debate will increase in intensity, because new biologic technologies have placed a huge number of new medications in the pipeline. They are undergoing clinical trials and offer promising, but expensive, additions to the pharmaceutical armamentarium.

In contrast to Americans, Canadians and other foreign nationals are purchasing prescription medications manufactured in the United States at about a 30 percent discount. The size of the problems is such that federal legislation is pending to permit importation of U.S. prescription drugs back into the United States. It is difficult to understand why selling at a higher price in the United States than in foreign countries is not considered predatory pricing that could be pursued under federal law.

Federal statutes should be adopted that even-handedly prevent drug companies from gaming the system to extend drug patents. Likewise, FDA should facilitate introduction of generic equivalents to reduce medication costs.

Physicians have little control over the price of medications, but their prescribing behaviors can significantly affect the cost of medications. The use of generic drugs and the prescribing of the cheaper of two equally efficacious medications can help contain the rising cost of medications. Likewise, physicians should resist being the first adopters of each new high-priced medication detailed by the "missionary sales force" of drug companies who offer small bribes of buying lunch for the office force, liberally dispense sample medications, and sponsor scientific meetings.

Health Promotion/Disease Prevention

As we have discussed in chapter II, managing the patient's entire health care needs takes a considerable investment in time and resources. The benefits and return on investment from these activities produce both short and long-term value. More money and effort should be devoted to these activities.

Stamping Out Disease

One societal value that has become inculcated in the community of physicians and patients is to do whatever is necessary to "stamp out disease." One has to raise the question, at what cost? Let's use an example to examine this issue. Prostate cancer is the most common cancer in men, with approximately 300,000-400,000 new cases per year and 35,000 deaths. In the vast majority of cases, prostate cancer is slow growing and occurs in elderly patients. In controlled studies, the 10-year crude survival rates for diagnosed prostate cancer are roughly the same with and without aggressive treatment, and less than 15 percent of patients diagnosed with prostate cancer actually die of the disease.

If a universal program were undertaken to screen for and treat prostate cancer, including rectal exam and PSAs at six-month intervals, repeated biopsies of the prostate, and aggressive medical and surgical management for all patients, it could consume up to 5 percent of all health care dollars. Similar scenarios can be painted for breast and colon cancer. There will always be a scarcity of health care dollars. How much is society willing to spend for one week, one month, or one year of survival benefit, the quality of which is compromised by aggressive treatment? At present, from a cost-effectiveness perspective, no adequate information exists to estimate a cost per quality of adjusted life year. This raises profound moral issues that will multiply as new scientific discoveries continue to emerge. This example highlights a need to look critically at cost-utility analysis and for health care policy experts to make tough choices based on sound data. Better standards need to be created on which to base clinical decisions.

There is a marked disparity in the amount of dollars spent on research for various high-profile diseases, such as AIDs, cancer, and heart disease. This discrepancy, which often does not reflect the incidence or prorated impact on society of the disease, is fueled by attention provided in the media, direct advertising to the health care consumer by pharmaceutical companies, and the trendy special interest groups in the "disease of the month competition." It seems inappropriate for high-profile celebrities without medical credentials to push special health interests because they are victims of certain diseases. This altruistic marketing distorts the allocation of health care dollars. A case in point is seen in prostate cancer, where testimonials from many public figures have irresponsibly pushed aggressive screening and treatment.

The practicing physician should be involved in balancing the use of scarce medical resources. Specialty societies and special interest groups must pull back from indorsing initiatives that lack compelling supportive data and metrics. This will help prevent distortions in the allocations of health care dollars.

Unwarranted Tests

There is considerable variation in the number of tests ordered by individual physicians. Some clinical reports suggest that between 50 and 80 percent of lab tests are unnecessary. Causes of inappropriate testing include:

- Lack of standardization of diagnostic critical pathways and algorithms.

- The belief that "failure to diagnose" could expose the physician to malpractice lawsuits (defensive medicine).

- Patient pressure on the doctor to fully investigate all signs and symptoms.

- ✦ The physician's compulsive behavior of thoroughness (the shotgun approach to diagnosis).

- ✦ The availability of sophisticated testing facilities and services in which the physician may have a monetary or other vested interest.

- ✦ Duplication of testing by PCPs and specialists.

- ✦ Test results that are inconclusive or erroneous and conflict with or cause uncertainty about the clinical diagnosis. It is difficult to accept the thesis that, if the lab result conflicts with the clinical picture, ignore the lab result.

- ✦ Ambiguous test reports that are written in a manner that mandates further testing for medical legal protection.

- ✦ Break down in communication and coordination between the treating physician and the testing facility.

- ✦ Tests that will not change the treatment plan regardless of their results but are considered a part of the routine work-up by the physician.

Huge savings can accrue if only appropriate tests are ordered. To eliminate waste, physicians must critically evaluate each ordered test. Does the test improve my capability to treat the patient? Does it provide critical answers about differential diagnosis? Is it a standard of practice and cost-effective? What are the benefits to the patient?

Treatment Venue

In general, when medical and surgical interventions are conducted safely in the office setting, it saves health care dollars. Transfer of care to the ED, outpatient center, or hospital operating room dramatically raises the cost by a multiple of four to ten.

We will use vasectomy as an example. The global fee for a vasectomy in the office under local anesthesia is approximately $400. When the procedure is transferred to the outpatient surgical venue, additional expenses are incurred, including scheduling and coordination of schedules, preoperative instruction, sign in and registration, ID bracelet, locker assignment with undressing, transportation via stretcher to the OR, pre-medication and starting the IV, operating room facility fee, charges for supplies and instrument packs, nurse monitoring of BP and pulse oximetry, postoperative check, completion of paperwork, and transportation from the OR. An average bill runs $2,000, even without general anesthesia. The surgeon's fee remains the same. Additionally his or her time is often used inefficiently when so many processes and schedules need to be coordinated.

Why aren't all vasectomies performed in physicians' offices?

✦ Patient preference to be sedated or to receive general anesthesia.

✦ The physician's lack of training in advanced cardiac life support (ACLS), which makes an adverse cardiac event more likely to be catastrophic in the office setting.

✦ Lack of resuscitation equipment.

✦ Inadequate assistants in the office.

✦ The appearance of being a high utilizer of hospital services and having a busy practice.

Appropriate use of the office for medical and surgical treatments has obvious advantages. It decreases costs and increases efficiency and productivity for the practicing physician. More offices should be configured to accommodate a wider range of office interventions.

Patterns of Practice

Utilization review programs that compile costs incurred by individual physicians for various CPT and ICD-9 codes produce graphs and statistics that reveal wide variation among physicians. Because physicians train in similar environments and have exposure to the same scientific literature, these variations probably do not relate directly to the shared reservoir of medical knowledge. We can speculate and list a few of the factors that might drive some differences in physicians' resource consumption.

✦ Incentives that directly relate to number of relative value units produced often drive utilization and affect patterns of practice, because the more services you provide the greater your income.

✦ It is a stimulant to physicians to feel that their time is fully engaged and in demand. To have a high hospital census and perform many surgical interventions often correlates with a physician's self-esteem.

- Being the early adopter brings the stimulus of mastering the new plus a higher level of visibility to professional colleagues. Moreover, newer procedure codes are usually reimbursed at a higher rate.

- Differing interpretation of the scientific literature and practice guidelines.

- The cost and utilization inefficiencies of inexperience and personal bias.

- Regional and local variability in standards of medical practice.

- I have this hammer (linear accelerator, new chemotherapeutic drug, fiber-optic endoscope, imaging center, etc) and am looking for nails to pound.

- Differing personality types with regard to compulsive and aggressive behaviors.

- Differing perspectives and philosophies between younger and older generations of physicians.

- Physician autonomy and freedom to select treatment modalities and innovate.

- The negligible impact that hospital utilization review and managed care guidelines have had in standardizing critical pathways.

The need for better defined guidelines that produce improved consistency and uniformity in cost-effective health care provision is obvious. These guidelines must come from collaboration, interaction, and consensus from groups of practicing physicians and result in an ideal standard of care. Physicians have the duty to come together to produce rational and realistic standards.

Medical Mistakes

During recent years a number of well-publicized studies have purported to show a high incidence of medical mistakes. Recently, the Institute of Medicine (IOM) found that between 44,000 and 98,000 preventable deaths occur yearly from medical errors. This equates to about $29 billion in medical expense, or close to 3 percent of all health care expenditures. Many more medical statistics have surfaced over the years that dismay physicians and communicate to the consumer that the system is unsafe and dangerous.

The findings from these studies are usually painted in sensational strokes by the media and are often extrapolated irresponsibly to general populations of patients. Moreover, using the clarity of hindsight afforded by the "retrospectocope," the anecdotal data are arbitrarily manipulated and massaged to achieve a point. That point is that the medical system is flawed and dangerous.

These attacks on the profession have been received with shocking passivity by the institutions representing organized medicine. Practicing physicians should be outraged by negative publicity that often misrepresents and distorts safeguards in the system.

Nevertheless, medical mistakes and sentinel events do occur. The physician community must recognize them, report them, learn from them, and take remedial steps to minimize the occurrence rate. Roughly 85-90 percent of medical mistakes are due to process errors and not lack of knowledge. Investment in electronic automation that streamlines processes, improves productivity, provides for cross-checking, eliminates illegible handwriting, creates better medical records, informs and educates patients, and improves connectivity between physicians and patients should decrease medical errors. In the process, health care dollars will be saved through decreased numbers of adverse events.

Summary

We have identified many of the major causes of high health care costs in the United States. None of the core causes lends itself to simple fiat solution. There is waste throughout the system. To speculate how much waste exists is pure conjecture. But we need to search for more answers to the question, Why does the United States spend 14 percent of its GDP, versus 8-10 percent for other developed countries, on health care without producing a measurably superior health status for its citizens? The physician has a pivotal role in understanding this incongruity and in providing the answers.

Understanding costs and micro-managing the costs in each encounter between physician and patient is a giant step toward reigning in costs and eliminating slack. The physician is critically positioned to be the agent for cost containment. If physicians don't shoulder the responsibility, outside players will continue to impose controls and legislate programs to reduce costs.

The amount of resources utilized by individual physicians to treat similar patient populations varies enormously. Using benchmarks of optimal resource utilization to achieve high-quality outcomes, studies have shown that some physicians expend two or even three times the number of health care dollars to treat the same illness. A case in point is C-section, where rates vary between eight and 35 percent. The data also suggest that the physician who over-utilizes or under-utilizes resources has inferior treatment outcomes. These variances need to be identified and remedial steps need to be taken to achieve optimal resource utilization. Physician education that focuses on the expenditure of health care dollars plus financial incentives tied to efficient resource consumption are two means to achieve this objective.

When confronted with statistics that suggest excessive resource use, physicians often respond that they have sicker patient populations. True, risk-adjusted severity of illness must be considered and factored into the mix. However, when a large database of ordinary charge data that has not been thoroughly "scrubbed" shows marked variation in dollars consumed by a physician to treat a similar population, it is usually a valid indicator of waste incurred by the physician.

Every physician can make a difference in health care costs and can be an agent for cost containment. Critically scrutinize your practice behaviors to see where you can make a difference. Physician independence will hinge upon our collective ability to justify every dollar spent on health care.

Chapter 4

Direct Contracting: Reclaiming the Franchise

Thirty years ago, in a time that physicians now perceive as the "golden era" of medicine, to practice medicine was uncomplicated. It was essentially a point-of-service cash business with only a modicum of third-party intervention and little or no intrusive oversight. Accountability was ensured by physician integrity and intellectual honesty. There was a genuine shortage of physicians and hospital beds, and health care consumed less than 10 percent of GDP. A physician's income directly correlated with how hard he or she wished to work. The physician community was respected, and the doctor/patient relationship involved a high level of trust. Office processes were straightforward, and on-the-job training for employees sufficed to achieve job mastery. The vast majority of physicians were soloists, and the physician was his or her own office manager. Most medical professionals considered marketing and advertising activities unethical. None of the above statements about medical practice hold true today. Physicians' Camelot has vanished.

Today, the community of physicians is under attack from all sides. The physician has been relegated to "provider status," as just one of the many players in the marketplace. Coupled with this loss of franchise, the physician community has been placed under the microscope. The integrity of physicians is questioned, and pervasive rules and regulations have been legislated to control health care. Intermediaries, who collectively control the purse strings, including federal and state government, MCOs, and employers, all push for increased oversight and accountability. There is excess capacity across all health care services. Competition and managed care have emerged as the cure for the ills of the health care system. Cost containment is the battle cry.

As one might expect, physician response to the new playing field has been generally unenthusiastic. Their token adjustment to the new demands attests to the resistance that most physicians feel toward the current medical environment. Often, physicians seem to focus their response exclusively on ways to maintain reimbursements and income levels. Unionization and collective bargaining, plus negotiating power and safety within large group practices, are some current strategies. However, heavy-handed tactics will not serve the long-term interests of the medical profession. It is too noble a profession to wrestle with competing interests for health care dollars. The general populace has little sympathy for the financial plight of physicians and other providers. The physician must command the high ground in the struggle to revolutionize the system.

In today's turbulent medical marketplace, perhaps the words that best describe the physician's feeling are "ambivalence" and "vulnerability." In general, most physicians would like to be left alone to care for patients. Fortunately or unfortunately, that compartmentalized and insulated luxury box is no longer an option for practicing physicians. If physicians wish to retain their independence, they must lead and manage a change process to rectify the many structural problems in the system that have produced repeated and lingering market failures. The community of physicians is the only player with the toolbox to fix the system.

In this chapter, we design a model that reshapes the marketplace by increasing physician influence and transferring power and choices to the patient. The goal is to enact a plan that:

✦ Makes MCO intermediaries extinct by empowering medical group practices to contract directly and successfully.

✦ Empowers physicians as managers and leaders who can build the infrastructure to manage patient populations, improve quality, contain costs, and administer health care plans.

✦ Uses control of patient information to underpin these activities.

The information age and the electronic revolution provide physicians the tools with which to manage and use information. Throughout America, automation and information control has profoundly changed the way companies do business. Tiers of intermediaries and administrators interposed between the customer and the business have been eliminated. Electronics are the heart of the management tools for a business to successfully market and sell directly to the customer. If physicians can come together to form large efficient medical organizations that offer a broad range of plans and choices, why shouldn't this hold true for the medical business?

MCOs, as intrusive intermediaries with a mission to harness physicians, have contained costs by decreasing reimbursements; limiting covered medical care services; cherry-picking younger, healthier populations; and mandating shorter hospital stays. Their success is directly proportional to the monetary stress imposed collectively on providers. But recent increases in health care costs suggest that the MCO model may no longer offer additional cost containment benefits. Reimbursements have been squeezed to the limit, and further savings must come from other initiatives. As a footnote, MCOs have produced virtually no documented evidence of improved quality of care received by the American public. Some commentators even suggest that MCOs have had a negative impact on the quality of care.

On average, MCOs consume 20-25 percent of health care premiums through administrative, marketing, and underwriting expense and profits. Do their services justify this high cost? What value-added service do they perform that justifies their interposition between providers and patients? In the '80s and early '90s, there may have been a need for a managed care entity or "organizer" to bring together the fragmented pieces of the medical landscape. Costs were out of control. Employers needed a better way to manage and predict costs. But is this true today?

In today's market, MCO administrative expense has become unnecessary baggage. Technology has given the physician the tools to manage the patient relationship and control patient information. Large physician groups have the financial resources to make the investment both in information systems and in hiring qualified technologists and executive managers. Physicians have developed more business savvy. A significant number have gone back to school to get MBA and MHA degrees or enrolled in courses such as those sponsored by the American College of Physician Executives. Many continuing medical education (CME) courses are devoted to practice management, group formation, and legal matters. The medical profession is tuning up for the business challenges ahead.

Ironically, the orientation toward management skills has occurred in response to the requirements of managed care. Physicians have been forced to game the system and position their practices to ensure inclusion in limited panels of doctors, maintain incomes, and procure necessary treatment for their patients. In many regions of the country MCOs have coerced doctors into forming group practices by excluding soloists from their HMO panels. This corralling of physicians is alleged to improve quality of care, but in reality it is designed to enhance MCO control and decrease administrative costs. Paradoxically, group formation and business know-how are the instruments by which physicians will achieve command.

Equipped with adequate information systems and a reservoir of physician executives, the community of physicians is positioned to eliminate intermediaries and have direct influence over the marketplace. Medical practices can be designed to administer population-based medicine and, in the process, restrain administrative and marketing expenses.

To restructure and reinvent medical organizations requires change that is driven by the physician. Some barriers to this change stem from personality and character traits shared by physicians.

- ✦ Physicians are very bright people on average; they initiate projects with great enthusiasm and have excellent conceptual vision. However, on psychological tests, they exhibit tendencies to be poor finishers and fall short in overall tenacity. With their scientific bent, physicians do not like ambiguity and expect quick results. Crafting new medical institutions is arduous and requires dogged persistence in overcoming a series of sticky problems. Organizational change introduces stress and uncertainty. Likewise, the work of reinventing the organization is often uncompensated and thankless.

- ✦ Remaking physician organizations is analogous to starting a new entrepreneurial business. It imposes financial and personal risk, and many physicians are risk averse.

- ✦ Physicians are accustomed to autonomy and independence. Some of them worry that computerization and group formation will dilute their authority and control. In the new framework, physicians must work collaboratively, let go of special agendas, overcome petty jealousies, and learn team dynamics. Information technology should be viewed as the workhorse to bring physicians together to manage the transformation.

- To reengineer the system, physicians must draw on outside expert assistance from highly paid and skilled administrators and technologists. Some physicians resist delegation to and empowerment of outside agents.

- Many physicians remain computer illiterate and are resistant to learning business skills.

- Under the current system, physician incomes are pegged directly to the number of relative value units (RVU) they generate. This emphasis on production line productivity encourages the physician to rush patients through the office encounter and to refer complex, time-consuming problems to specialists. This explicit time clock approach to medical care negatively affects the patient relationship and the quality of holistic care. Pay formulas will need revision to overcome this deficiency.

- Finally, physicians must appreciate and address the anxiety of staff members who may fear layoffs and job modifications as a result of the reengineering process.

These are generalizations. There exists a cadre of well-qualified physician leaders and managers who are eager to lead the revolutionary change process.

An Administration Model for Direct Contracting: Crafting the New Marketplace

Thus far, we have proposed three broad change initiatives: patient-focused strategies, managing the patient relationship, and control of health care costs. These change models will produce the internal reengineering of medical practices to become efficient and effective entities in the provision of health care services. Each of these initiatives can be viewed as forming one of three integrated columns that support a platform for successful direct contracting. This practice evolution into a complete business entity that manages all aspects of health care and information is now positioned to exercise its revolutionary and appropriate role in the medical marketplace. It is poised to form effective external alliances to offer a comprehensive package of health care services to the consumer. Financial control and decision making are returned to physicians and patients.

Having stated the central thesis, the author admits to having no "special" knowledge or a crystal ball. The medical environment has a mind-boggling array of strong players, each with different perspectives and agendas. It is hard to predict how e-commerce and e-healthcare will affect the consumer and the marketplace. Future federal and state legislation and the direction of the Medicare and Medicaid programs cannot be forecast with certainty. The influence of hospitals and managed care organizations will not be conceded to physicians without a fight. Pharmaceutical companies will seek to maintain their profit margins. Academic medical centers will continue to explore ways to ensure adequate funding and in all likelihood will increasingly compete with the private sector for patients. Many more unknowns exist that complicate any model that reinvents the system.

Despite the erratic influences that fragment the system of health care, the practicing physician must look at ways to reform the system to better carry out the mission of service to humanity. They must not be passive observers and followers who await directions from other players. They must be proactive, create a collective vision, and revolutionize the system to make it more user-friendly to the patient. This may sound like fancy rhetoric, but the author believes that physicians can and must take charge of the change process.

Physician behavior is often characterized as staunchly independent and autonomous. It is often repeated that trying to organize and regiment physicians is like trying to "herd cats." Certainly, when outside forces try to disenfranchise and control physicians with meddlesome macro-managed initiatives, this description of physician behavior is fairly accurate. However, committed physicians working together with a common mission are a formidable force. Their creativity and independence are highly positive traits for crafting an optimal medical system. Physicians need to stop whining about the way things are, actively lay the ground work for how things can and should be, and work toward that goal. Physicians possess the skills, knowledge, and abilities to create a medical system that better serves the patient consumer of health care.

Obviously, a direct contracting plan by physician organizations will not quickly replace current payment systems. Each local and regional market has unique characteristics and differing degrees of managed care penetration. Reinventing medical organizations takes time, and maneuvering the medical marketplace behemoth is like steering a large floating iceberg.

But by giving improved options to consumers, the new physician model for direct contracting will demonstrate its value by capturing a larger share of the market. The displacement of managed care organizations will be achieved through the competitive advantages derived from Independence Day strategies.

To transfer financial control back to physicians and patients, let's first discuss some of the basic structural requirements for a large medical group practice to directly contract. Then we will analyze additional factors necessary for the system to fit together and become operational.

Structural Requirements

✦ Simple Organizational Structure

– An administrative entity similar to a third-party administrator (TPA) that manages costs but, in most instances, does not seek to be an insurance company or hold an HMO license. In order to compete in some markets, the "administrator" may need the capability to contract with some degree of risk sharing with strategic partners. Flexibility will be a key element for an administrator to accommodate market conditions.

– Offers several plans with varying copayments for treatment, carve-outs of uncovered services, and provision for out-of-area coverage.

– Assists employers and other group purchasers in developing self-funded or alternate funding style plans. Informs uninsured individuals about direct enrollment and the benefits afforded by medical savings accounts and tax incentives available for self-insurance.

– A separate profit center structure that is an independent contractor to or a strategic business unit (SBU) of the medical group practice.

✦ A format that embodies some of the features of gatekeeping responsibility for the PCP but gives enrollees direct access to a wide range of specialty care. This avoids duplication of services and allows more cost-effective management of critical pathways.

+ A plan without physician risk-sharing provisions, capitation (fixed payment per enrollee), or other incentives that encourage the physician to withhold care. More appropriately, physician incentives would be linked to measurements such as patient satisfaction scorecards, quality of care standards, and efficient resource utilization. These positive motivators institutionalize the physician as a patient advocate.

  Some observers might challenge the assumption that the good intentions of physicians will contain costs without the restraints of capitation and risk sharing. To respond, it can be stated that the medical group has a better incentive system. Pay formulas for its physicians are linked to patterns of practice and resource utilization. The physician who wastes resources when compared with his or her peers in treating similar populations of patients is penalized. Recall the fact that physicians direct 80-85 percent of health care expenditures. For the most part, waste in the system relates to misuse of resources. An incentive tied to practice patterns positively focuses the physician on effective behaviors, unlike the strict monetary incentives of capitation that focus a physician's behavior on short-changing the patient.

+ Administrative efficiency that is enabled by control and access to all patient information generated by the medical group and its strategic partners.

+ A three-pronged program for physician education on economic issues and costs.

  – Gathering and disseminating information about actual medical care costs.

  – A committee to evaluate cost/utility ratios of conventional treatments and interventions plus new investigative technologies.

  – Medication evaluation and crafting a formulary that factors in costs.

+ A continuous quality improvement (CQI) program that goes beyond token parameters. Optimally, the program would include three or four physicians working collaboratively in their areas of expertise to draft critical pathways and algorithms. Experience attests to this small group process as being most efficient and effective in defining guidelines and standards of medical care. This is in contrast to outside health care organizations, with their convoluted evidence-based medicine (EBM) standards, that produce statistical certainty and precision that is not easily applied to clinical practice. Their explicit clinical practice guidelines (CPG) are often incomplete and have limitations in conceptual, methodological, and practical terms. Within the framework of a group practice, physicians can directly influence the behavior of other physicians. An interactive process in the group can result in significantly less variation in patterns of practice. Moreover, with the coalescence of large medical groups, there is a natural tendency for subspecialization within the framework of a center of excellence or a "focused factory" concept. Horizontal integration of practices to achieve scope and quality in this manner is a cost-saving, efficient strategy.

✦ For direct contracting, the core medical group must be large and provide the capacity to administer to the health care needs of the full range of enrollee groups. Most large employers prefer a large number of physicians for their employees' selection. The optimal size of a single- or multispecialty group in a large metropolitan area might equal 400-600 physicians. Broad geographic coverage is pivotal. Strategic alliances with other medical groups to fill in the gaps in physician coverage might be necessary. Moreover, extensive networking with hospitals, ancillary service providers, and other providers would be a requirement. Negotiated contracts can flesh out the plan and provide additional ways to manage costs.

✦ The new enterprise will need adequate capitalization as a start-up venture. Because the administrative entity could be a separate strategic business unit (SBU) of the group practice or be subcontracted to an independent agency, many ways to finance the initial capitalization can be considered. These include outside venture and angel capital, bank loans, assessment of group members, and joining fees. An adequate information technology infrastructure and qualified managers are a prerequisite.

✦ A comprehensive business and marketing plan that includes a financial pro forma should be written.

Operational Considerations

Employers with benefit plans view health care coverage for their employees as a cost of doing business. They need to know how to budget for this expense. To meet these requirements, a health care administrative plan with self-funding or alternate funding would need to produce realistic cost projections. Projections are enabled through use of the informational databases provided by the group practice and employee personnel files. With enrollee groups of 1,000 or more people, realistic predictions should be achievable. These information resources can produce experience-rated estimates and prospectively factor in the health-risk profiles of employees. Community rating profiles (average health care expense across the entire community of enrollees) could be used in selected circumstances along side utilization data from the group practice.

Additional opportunities for direct contracting exist with the 40+ million uninsured persons in the United States, and with health cooperatives, group health purchasing associations, unions, and so on. With individual or groups of enrollees, the administrative body could share cost efficiencies and discounts through a direct or consolidated sign-up program.

Previously, we detailed the broad range of information compiled when managing the patient relationship. This comprehensive database of patient information affords the medical group the ability to extract, estimate, and report on the cost of caring for identified patient populations. The practice's utilization experience and medical risk profiling data, plus experience-rated hospital, ancillary service, pharmacy utilization, and specialty care data, would be used to compile and produce experience-rated costs and analysis. Modern information technology makes precise tracking of costs achievable. Each item and activity are costed on the basis of both the supply and the demand sides of the ledger and are extrapolated to targeted patient populations to produce reliable figures for the employer.

The program would expand the definition of treating physician to give the patient direct access to a wide range of medical specialists. In each medical group, the model would need to be tailored to accommodate the mix of physicians. Many medical specialists, such as gastroenterologists, pulmonologists, cardiologists, dermatologists, rheumatologists, ophthalmologists, and nephrologists, provide long-term care for chronic conditions. Ongoing direct access to these specialists supports continuity of care and captures cost efficiencies. Family practitioners, internists, obstricians/gynecologists, and pediatricians would continue to be "primary treating physicians," and the information systems of all "specialty" practices would need to interface with the information system of the "treating physician." As a result, the primary treating physician becomes the repository for all patient information to be shared with the medical practice administrator.

Reimbursements for the treating physician and selected specialists would be on a fee-for-service basis, with bonuses tied to the incentives discussed previously.

Other operational features include:

- Requests for proposal (RFPs) would be solicited from specialty groups. Specialists would initially be contracted on a capitated basis. Payments would be pegged to Medicare rates until satisfactory experience-rating data became available.

- The third-party administrator model would require strategic relationships to provide ancillary services. Laboratory services could be contracted on a negotiated fee-per-patient basis. Routine and interventional radiology services could be directed to selected facilities, such as imaging centers or hospital departments, that would negotiate discounted professional and facility fees. Their information systems would need to directly interface with the information system of the medical group practice to permit entry of testing results and charge data. Other services, such as physical therapy and nuclear medicine, would be partnered in a similar fashion.

- Contracts with hospitals for inpatient services would be negotiated through the same process used by managed care organizations. Hospital rates would be set on a per diem rate or discounted basis, with a goal to achieve "most favored nation" or best rate status. The use of outpatient surgical centers owned by entities other than hospitals could be used to lower facility fees.

- Special relationships could be formed with pharmacy chains and mail order drug houses to manage pharmacy benefit programs. The cost savings would flow directly to enrollees. Unlike the approach taken by MCOs, the formulary would be developed on the basis of drug efficacy and the direct cost to the consumer rather than on year-end rebates from pharmaceutical houses for bulk usage.

- Carve outs and stop loss insurance could be utilized to contain risk for group plans. Coverage for services such as chiropractic, neonatal intensive care, organ transplantation, experimental therapies, and plastic surgery, plus items such as durable medical equipment and life-style medications, could be added or subtracted, depending on the group purchaser's choice.

This snapshot provides a bare bones framework for a complicated process. In reality, getting all partners and subcontractors to negotiate on the same page and interface electronically is a formidable task. However, if the medical group, by virtue of its large size, has considerable "buyer power" and influence, the negotiations to round out the plan and fill in the gaps can be satisfactorily accomplished. This must occur if the group practice plans to directly contract, regain economic control, and give the patient better choices.

Direct contracting by medical groups is a logical strategy that overcomes many of the market failures inherent in traditional managed care. It eliminates middleman waste and uses patient information to improve quality of care and contain health care costs. Although not unique, this plan affords a template for organized physicians to develop, control, and drive the system. It bypasses third-party payers, introduces direct price competition among medical groups, gives patients more choices, and supports improved quality of care. The physician becomes both a manager and patient advocate on the road to improved managed care.

Earlier in the chapter, we noted how the three integrated column model supports direct contracting. In return, direct contracting reinforces the efforts and returns from each of the three support legs. They fit together as an integrated package to become the "one-stop shopping" destination for the consumer of health care.

This administrative model is just one of many potential models for a group practice to market directly to the consumer. Many creative and innovating approaches can be used. The goal remains the same; physicians regain the franchise.

Chapter 5

The Reengineering Process

Sadly for some, medicine is no longer a mom-and-pop business anchored entirely to the doctor/patient relationship. It is a big business and is being subjected to all the forces of change, scrutiny, and tampering that are seen in contemporary America. Physicians must meet this challenge with revolutionary determination to take command.

We have covered many of the general themes and paradigm shifts necessary to transform medical practices into high performance, integrated business entities to support the physician's reemergence as the leader in the transformation of health care. Table 5-1, page 94, contrasts the old with the new.

Briefly, large integrated medical groups provide the means for capital formation, resource development, and specialization of personnel. The new medical practice responds to the patient's wants and needs by offering a supermarket of health care services in an environment of exemplary service. Electronic automation streamlines business processes, facilitates open connectivity between all stakeholders, and supports the option of a paperless office. Patient and practice information is collected and managed to improve quality of care, support models for direct contracting, and handle the administrative activities of population-based medical care. Physicians and patients together assume

Table 5-1. Medical Practice Transormation

Old	New
Independent Groups	Consolidated Groups
Limited Resources	Patient Supermarket
Paper Transactions	Electronic Automation
Paper Chart	Paperless Office
Treatment	Exemplary Service
Intermediary Control	Physician and Patient Control
Fragmented Data	Information Control
Limited Interactions	Open Connectivity
Physician Authority	Physician Responsibility

responsibility for forging a partnership in health care. To recapture the franchise, medical organizations are reinvented.

To transform medical practices into outstanding service and administrative entities in the rapidly changing information age is a formidable task. The many profound change models outlined in this book prompt physicians to ask where to begin and in what sequence to focus their efforts. Figure 5-1, page 95, gives an overview of the logical steps in the reengineering process. Practice enhancement efforts are divided into two major classifications. The first classification is internal to the practice and builds the infrastructure and platform that support the second classification—external activities of strategic partnerships and direct contracting. The flow chart is a road map of increasing medical practice capabilities. Each successive step builds on the previous step.

The author has often seen medical group practices attempt to navigate the road map in the reverse direction. They start with strategic partnerships and risk contracting before the internal infrastructure is in place to support such relationships. This is a consistent formula for dysfunctional partnering and financial disappointment. A medical group practice must have its internal house in order before undertaking major external projects.

Figure 5-1.

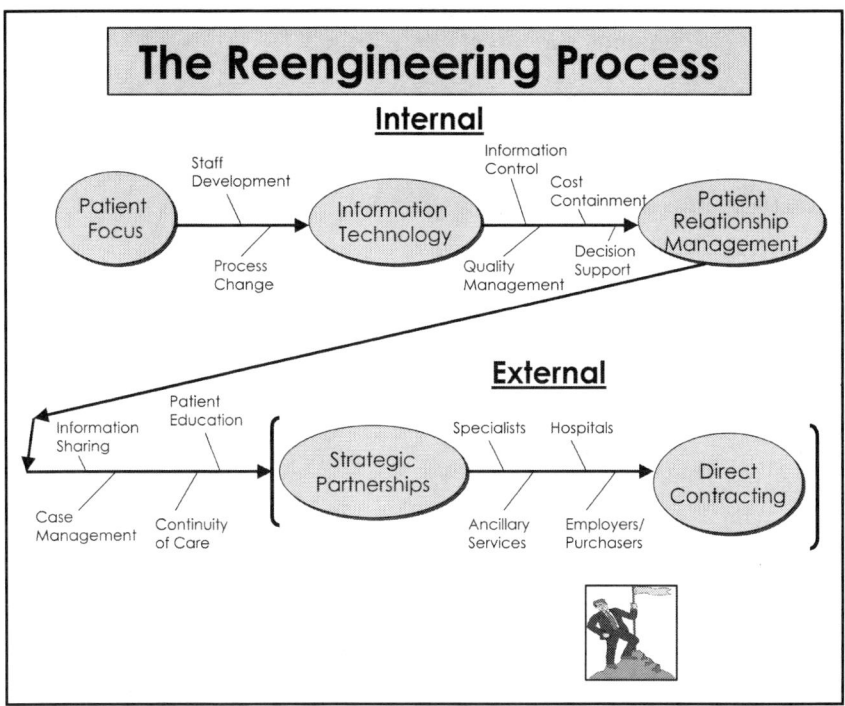

The critical first step and the foundation for practice enhancement is patient service. When medical practices transform into exemplary service organizations they better fulfill the critical medical mission to serve. A cadre of loyal patients garnered through outstanding service supports practice growth and profitability. Moreover, "patient-focused strategies" are cost saving and survival strategies for medical practices.

Once the service ethic is embedded in the organization, the medical practice is positioned to exploit the benefits of proactively managing the patient relationship. Appropriate use of information technology enables a practice to become a streamlined business organization with efficient processes. The relationship with the patient is leveraged into a partnership in health care. Information control and the capability to analyze and manage costs support external strategic partnerships and direct contracting of medical services.

Medical practices should avoid strategic plans that put the "cart before the horse." The horse that pulls the medical organization relates to the components of internal practice improvement. Only after this engine is in place can a medical practice successfully fill the cart with strategic partnerships and direct contracting.

The blueprint of excellence detailed in the book supports a revolution in physicians' role in the medical marketplace. The strategies and tactics outlined are empowerment vehicles for physicians. They must lead the transformation and, as a result, regain their independence.

Appendix A
Value Mapping Worksheets: How Does Your Practice Stack Up?

Convenient Appointment

Difficulty in getting a convenient appointment is a frequently voiced patient complaint (figure A-1, page 98).

Patient's Perspective

It is frequently observed that, when a doctor calls another doctor to make a personal appointment, he or she is given preferential treatment and scheduled expeditiously. Doctors do not realize how difficult it is to make an appointment at a convenient time from a layperson's perspective. How often do patients have to wait a month to be seen for routine visits or a week for more urgent matters?

To engender patient confidence that they can receive timely medical care, they must have appropriate access to the doctor. Although some symptoms may seem trivial to the physician, to the patient they are usually perceived as urgent matters. The frustration and prolonged worry caused by having to wait many days to "get in" is a common source of dissatisfaction.

The Cause of the Problem

+ The practice's volume of patients is too large to squeeze everybody in.

| *Independence Day*

Figure A-1.

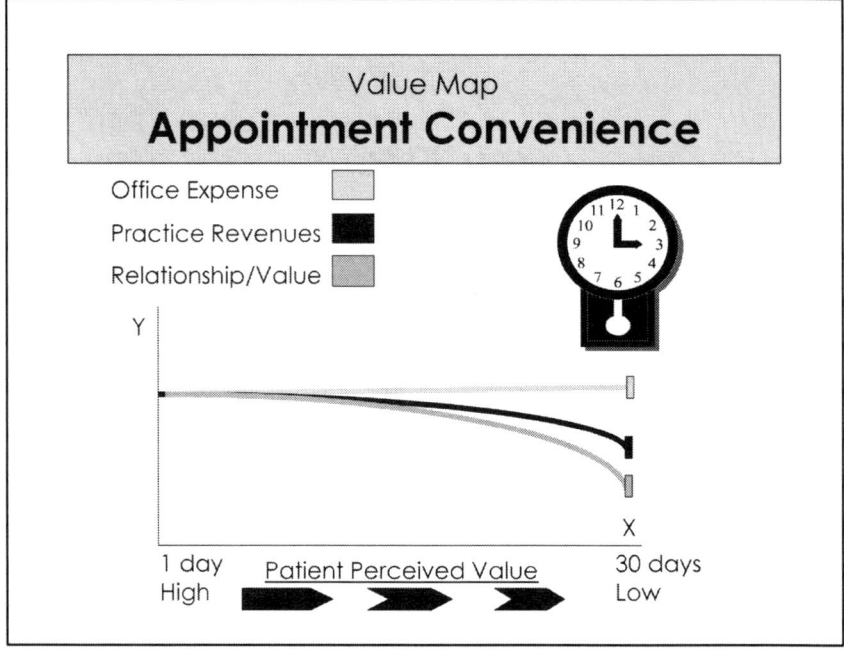

- Doctors have set limits on how hard or how many hours they wish to work.

- Staff members have set limits on how hard or how many hours they wish to work.

- The physician uses his or her time inefficiently. He or she may consistently arrive late or have too many distracting outside activities.

- The physician is unwilling to delegate mundane care functions to the staff. These functions consume physician time that could be freed up to handle a larger volume of patients.

- It builds the physician's self-esteem to know that patients are waiting in line to be seen.

Solutions

Analysis of appointment delays may need to be determined subjectively, because first it needs to be determined if it is creating a problem with quality of care. Are urgent and emergency medical needs being met?

What is the level of patient dissatisfaction?

The solutions may vary, but this problem lends itself to solution because delays in scheduling an appointment are usually a reflection of a busy practice. Full employment of a physician's time is one of the hallmarks of a successful practice.

- Recruit a new associate.
- Design tactics in a group practice to off-load excessive patient loads to an associate.
- Expand office hours to accommodate one or two more patients per day and get caught up with the patient backlog. The increased revenue generated falls directly to the bottom line, because the variable costs of extending office hours are minimal.
- Train your employees to be "physician extenders." Delegate to them all activities that they are competent to perform.
- Look at a range of ideas to improve efficiency, such as electronic scheduling programs and e-scheduling.
- Craft guidelines that focus on realistic targets that minimize the delay in receiving an appointment.
- Provide insight into and training in the art of appointment scheduling for the staff.
- Design a more flexible schedule with slots for urgent problems and drop ins.

Costs

To see patients as soon as possible and to shorten the interval to be seen does not increase office expense. Depending only on the condition and the patient, doctors spend a predictable amount of time with each patient. Seeing a patient sooner rather than later does not consume additional physician time.

It is readily apparent that, as the interval between setting up an appointment and being seen increases, practice revenues decrease. The bottom line takes a big hit. Why?

- Patients get well spontaneously and cancel appointments.

Independence Day

- The no show ratio increases.
- Patients defect, go elsewhere, and switch doctors.
- Patients lose faith in their ability to access care.

It may be reassuring for the doctor to feel he or she is busy, but when it takes too long to get in to see the doctor, it has a negative long-term effect on a practice. The testimonial from a patient who has to wait a month usually goes like this, "I like the doctor but I can't get in to see him." Would you select that physician for your care?

The majority of patient satisfaction studies report equal or better patient satisfaction scores for nurse practitioners when compared to physicians. The main areas in which nurse practitioners score higher are active listening, amount of advice, support, and thoroughness. The pay for a nurse practitioner or a physician extender is a fraction of that for the doctor, so it makes financial sense to use them more extensively. Their use is a powerful tool to enhance a physician's productivity and revenue stream.

Finally, if a practice receives 40 calls per day for new appointments and only 30 patients are seen per day, what happens to the other 10 patients? How do they fall through the cracks? What is the economic impact on the practice, and what if just one more patient were seen per day? Do the numbers!

Billing Errors

Patient's Perspective (figure A-2, page 101)

Consumers of health care either directly or indirectly pay high premiums for their health insurance. This may lead them to expect comprehensive first-dollar insurance coverage. Often, they have not read the insurance booklet that details carve outs, copayments, and uncovered services. To receive a bill may violate their expectations and cause anxiety. This often prompts many phone calls from patients for clarification of bills after the billing cycle.

Practices should take steps to ensure that patients understand office policies concerning billing and the limits of their insurance coverage. To receive an inaccurate statement or charges for services not performed causes resentment and anger. Likewise, a slow or defensive response to

Figure A-2.

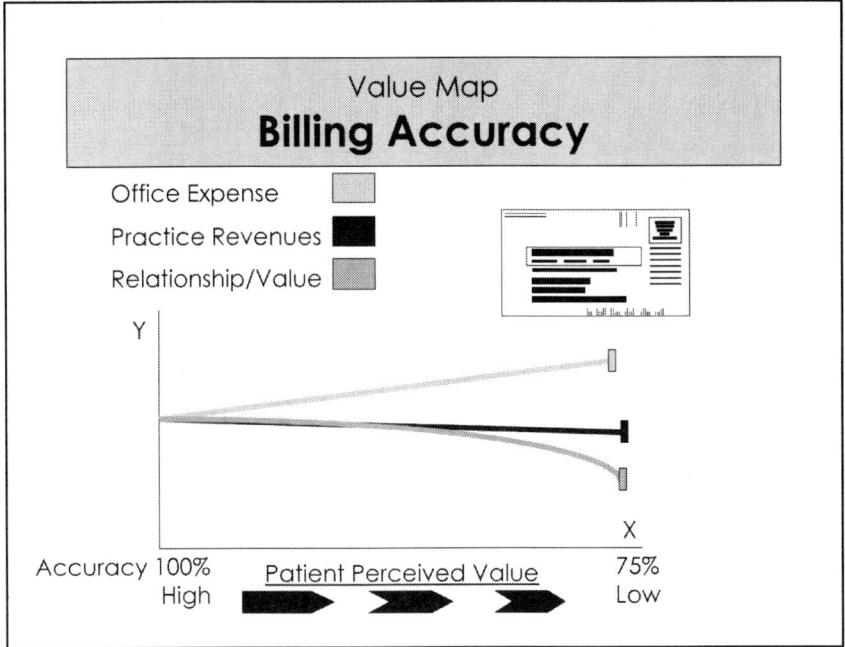

patients' inquiries or challenges causes patients to view the practice as indifferent to their needs.

To Uncover the Problem

Fielding irate calls about bills is an unpleasant task for office staff. The office manager usually has first-hand knowledge about the existence of a problem. He or she can provide information about the month-to-month increases or decreases in the number of calls related to charges that require a turnaround or an apology from office staff.

Causes of the Problem

+ Inaccurate entry of charges on routing slips. The physician entry may be inaccurate because of slip design, carelessness, lack of coding expertise, or an excess of redundant codes. Often, physicians in the same practice use different codes for the same condition or procedure.

+ Delayed entry of charge data into the computer system if the physician is not available to clarify charges when codes are confusing.

- Inexperienced billing personnel or MSO support billing specialists.

- Computer software that is not user-friendly and requires double entry of billing data.

- MCO denials and letters sent to the patient from the MCO that question a physician's charges. These letters are a frequent cause of patient inquiries and often undermine the credibility of the doctor.

- Faulty tracking of explanations of benefits (EOBs) that causes duplicate bills to be sent and untracked revenues to "fall through the cracks."

- Discovery of lost unbilled charges and insurance denials of coverage charges that are sent to the patient many months after the service is performed. The patient is often surprised, embarrassed, and angered by these late bills.

- The lack of a standard policy to write off charges. This problem sometimes relates to a breakdown in communication with contracted billing specialists.

- Lack of a standardized procedure to manage insurance issues for patients.

- Different billing software programs in separate office locations in a group practice that do not seamlessly interface.

Solutions

- Demonstrate the benefits of accurate coding to the physician. Smooth out the process of transferring data from the routing slip into the computer. Consider an EMR program that interfaces with the billing software to facilitate accurate coding and eliminate duplicate data entry. Discuss ways to improve accuracy.

- Standardize the billing process across all office locations.

- Review office policies and procedures concerning billing, and look for ways to streamline the process.

- Evaluate efficiency and ease of use of the billing software. Replace, if necessary, or even evaluate the benefits of outsourcing this function.

- Set a goal of 100 percent billing accuracy and periodically measure results by monitoring the number of complaints.

✦ Strive to send out the bills within 14 days of the date of the service. On the invoice, print the name and telephone number of the person to call if there are questions.

✦ Standardize the process of writing off uncollectables and closely follow the 30-, 60-, and 90-day accounts receivable. If there is no response to three bills and two alerts that state the account is overdue, in all probability you are not going to get paid and further statements just waste postage. Turning delinquent bills over to a collection agency rarely produces significant returns and often further alienates the patient. It should be reserved only for flagrant cases.

Even with a first-class billing system, an office will receive a flurry of patient calls after the billing cycle. The goal is to minimize the number and to have in place a process for quick response and friendly resolution of patient challenges. A quick turnaround is often instrumental in producing increased patient loyalty.

Costs

Each incorrect bill may cause a denial from a third-party payer. Any unjustified or incorrect claim may lead to the need for refilling, calls from upset patients, patient defections, and patient refusals to pay.

A flawed billing process increases office expense because of:

✦ Wasted time, and the expense of sending duplicate bills.

✦ Time necessary to track a large number of delinquent accounts and unpaid balances.

✦ Aggravating turnaround calls for office personnel.

✦ Lost revenues.

✦ Threat of third-party payer review of the practice.

✦ Collection agency expense.

Access the Physician both Day and Night

Patient's Perspective (figure A-3, page 104)

Phone access to the physician is vital for the patient. A timely call back or taking calls when received during regular office hours for routine

Figure A-3.

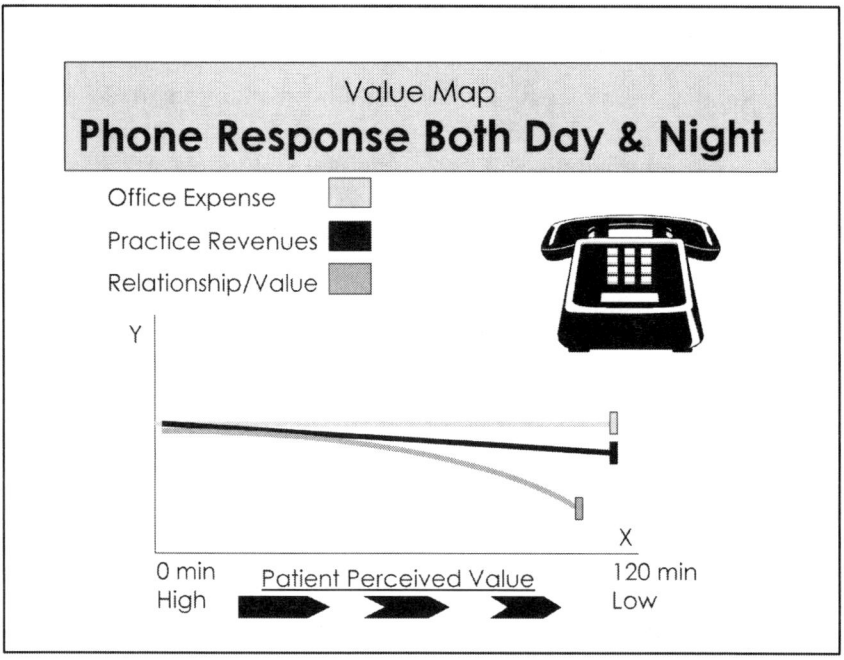

matters delights patients. The physician or his or her coverage must respond to emergencies and serious problems at all hours. Lack of appropriate response undermines patients' confidence in accessing health care and may cause them to go elsewhere for their medical care.

To Identify the Problem

✦ When the physician cannot be reached, patient defection to other providers may be immediate, with no voicing of the complaint. The office manager may be unaware of any problem.

✦ When phone access problems are discussed, both physician and staff may deny that a problem exists and place blame on outside coverage, the answering service, and faulty equipment.

✦ A physician may harbor negative feelings toward certain patients and rationalize his or her lack of response by saying that it takes too much time and is not worth the effort.

✦ Patient satisfaction surveys can usually reveal this problem if a question about phone access is included.

- ✦ Query the answering service about the number of patients who call after hours because their calls to the medical practice were not returned during regular office hours.

- ✦ Have the phone company track the number of busy signals.

Causes of the Problem

- ✦ An office staff that is not adequately trained to realistically screen and prioritize calls and put urgent ones directly through to the doctor.

- ✦ An answering service that does not filter and prioritize calls and does not consistently know how to reach the doctor.

- ✦ Poor coordination of coverage between physicians in the same or other practices.

- ✦ Unwillingness of a covering doctor to take overriding responsibility for a colleague's patients when the colleague is out of town or off call.

- ✦ A mind-set that the doctor works 9 to 5.

- ✦ Incorrect phone numbers.

- ✦ The bad habit of delaying the return of "nuisance calls" because of their inconvenience.

- ✦ Lack of a cell phone, pager or other electronic means to directly contact a physician.

Solutions

- ✦ Increase physicians' awareness concerning the importance of access.

- ✦ Improve communication between covering physicians, plus carefully coordinate on-call schedules between offices.

- ✦ Define for the staff the boundaries of responsibility for filtering calls and refilling prescriptions. Develop criteria for calls that should be immediately directed to the doctor.

- ✦ Periodically review the service provided by the after-hours answering service. A random "mystery call" from a staff member to the answering service can be used to evaluate courtesy and response. In chapter

II we discussed the advantages to a large group practice of maintaining a 24-hour "call center" to manage the interface with patients.

✦ Patient satisfaction survey questions that ask the patient to evaluate access to and response from the doctor and to offer suggestions.

✦ Instructive materials and wellness books that provide guidelines for when a patient should or should not call the doctor on an urgent basis.

✦ Adequate communication devices, such as car phones, pagers, and Web-enabled digital devices.

✦ Complete physician profile cards to assist emergency department physicians in treating the physician's patients. These sheets should contain the list of physicians to whom the doctor refers patients, indicate whether the primary physician wishes to be notified before or after treatment, and provide guidelines for follow-up care.

✦ In the schedule, create dedicated time periods in which the doctor returns routine phone calls. A goal for phone response should be 20 minutes for office staff and no more than one hour for physicians.

Costs

Timely physician response is very reassuring to the patient, and it decreases transaction costs for the practice. The benefits include:

✦ Quick response creates confident patients and eliminates the phone hassle for the patient.

✦ Repeated calls-ins and callbacks are minimized, and fewer loose ends remain to be dealt with at the finish of office hours. Moreover, it eliminates uncertainty about the nature of an unanswered call that may cause concern for the doctor and staff.

✦ A higher percentage of emergency problems are recognized and proactively dealt with early in the day at a propitious time for admission to the hospital and sophisticated testing. When a patient needs urgent specialty care, it facilitates scheduling and testing.

✦ The physician does not have to apologize for being unavailable.

✦ Prescription purchase to initiate treatment is expedited.

✦ The office staff has less difficulty in contacting patients who have

Figure A-4.

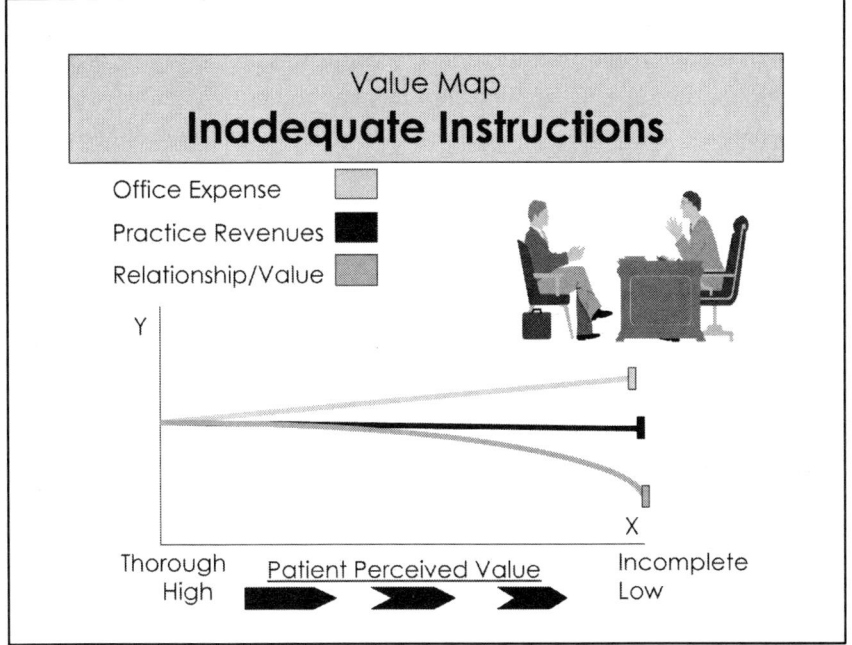

called within the hour, because they are more likely to be in the same place.

✦ Timely phone response is a risk management initiative that prevents serious problems from going unrecognized.

One caveat is warranted. Some patients persistently abuse the open phone door. Some may even want their medical care exclusively provided at no cost by phone. These difficult patients may need to be counseled about abuse of the phone and in some instances "fired" from a practice. However, placing a slow phone response barrier to frustrate this type of behavior is not a suitable solution; all it does is create angry defectors who plug into their social circle and unmarket your practice.

Inadequate Instruction

Patient's Perspective (figure A-4, above)

Individuals other than medical professionals have insufficient knowledge to navigate alone through the medical maze of diagnosis, testing, and treatment. Patients are often anxious and insecure about health matters. The dependent role they must assume in seeking medical care is often a source of emotional conflict. This tension can result in patients' hearing only what they want to hear and not the necessary information given in instructions. Thus, instructions need to be painstakingly provided. Repetition and reassurance may help ensure complete understanding. Thorough understanding is the centerpiece of patient compliance.

To Identify the Problem

✦ Examine the office process by which the patient receives information. Do the physician, the medical assistant, and front office personnel work together as a reinforcing team to ensure that instructions are thorough and completely understood?

✦ Record the number of phone calls received from patients seeking clarification of instructions.

✦ Track the number of tests ordered and procedures scheduled that were not carried out because of patient confusion about instructions. Record the number of tests that need rescheduling month to month as an indicator.

✦ On patient satisfaction surveys, ask if the doctor answered all questions and whether instructions were understood.

Causes of the Problem

✦ Patient anxiety and unfamiliarity with medical matters and medical jargon.

✦ Physician and staff assumed too much and did not devote enough time to instructing the patient.

✦ Lack of printed instructions for the patient to take home.

✦ Instructions were not repeated, and patient was not asked if they were fully understood.

✦ Instructions were too complicated or given in medical terms that were ambiguous.

✦ Mentally or physically challenged patient.

Solutions

✦ If the patient did not follow the plan of prescribed treatment, the physician should seek an explanation at the time of return visit. Did it relate to the instruction process, and, if so, how can the process be improved?

✦ At the end of the encounter, the receptionist or the medical assistant should ask the patient if all instructions are fully understood and take remedial steps if they are not.

✦ Repetition of instructions with emphasis placed on key points.

✦ Provide printed materials and computer-generated instructions to take home, supplemented as necessary by tailored, handwritten notes.

✦ Discuss treatment plans with attendants or family members who come with the patient.

✦ Have the staff schedule appointments for outside testing, and instruct the testing facility to convey additional information to the patient.

✦ If the patient is referred to specialists, call and make the appointment. Provide salient patient information along with the reason for referral via e-mail, fax, telephone, or handwritten note. Make certain the patient has the address and phone number of the specialist, and encourage him or her to report back after the visit to discuss the experience and receive further instructions.

✦ Send reminder notices that can be automated by computer, and make calls to make certain the patient knows about follow-up appointments and tests.

✦ Send computer-assisted personalized form letters to the patient that summarize the most recent encounter, testing results, and treatment objectives.

✦ Make postoperative follow-up calls to check on the condition of the patient and to answer questions.

✦ Have the patient write down a list of questions before seeing the doctor. These questions are more likely to be answered and, in return, the response is more likely to be understood.

Figure A-5.

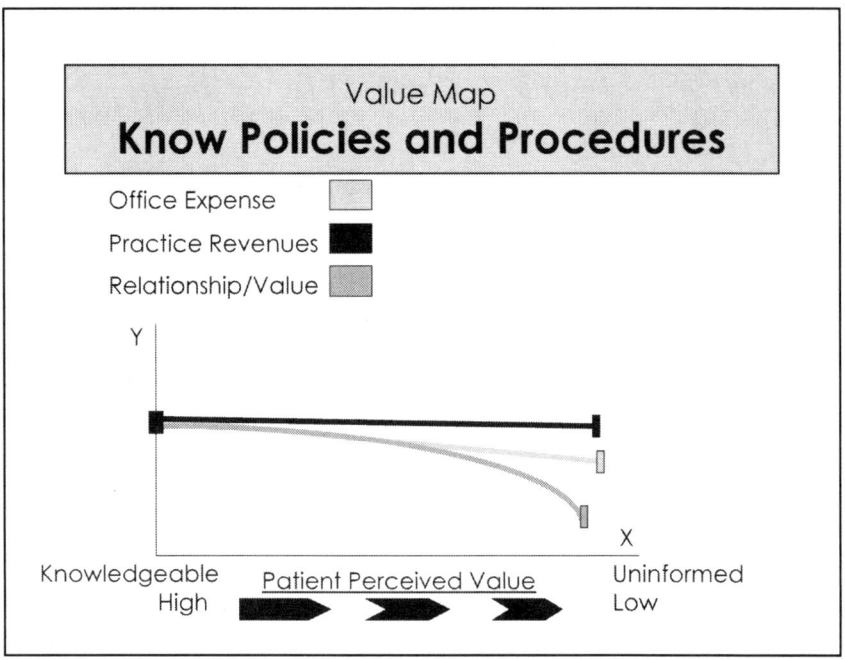

Costs

The time invested in ensuring complete understanding of instructions decreases the number of follow-up calls seeking clarification of routine instructions. Compliance, continuity of care, no shows, and quality of care are all improved. The number of patients needing rescheduling of tests decreases. Full patient understanding builds confidence in and comfort with the physician and the program of treatment. A medical practice should take steps to minimize the complaint that "the Doctor did not take the time to explain." Additionally, thorough instructions are a part of every physician's risk management program.

Known Policies, Procedures and General Practice Information

Patient's Perspective (figure A-5, above)

The more knowledge a patient has about an office's policies and procedures as well as general practice information, the higher his or her comfort level with interactions with the medical practice. Sampling of pertinent information include handling of insurance, hours of operation, return of phone calls, renewal of prescriptions, membership and participation in insurance products, acceptance of new patients, practice ownership, charge cards accepted, services provided, hospital staff privileges, key employees, health maintenance program, and physician qualifications. General knowledge about a practice instills familiarity and ease in the relationship between the patient and the practice. It minimizes the number of calls seeking answers to routine question.

On a very positive note, it delights most patients to know all about their doctors. This enables them to share this knowledge as well as their illnesses with their friends. This "grapevine" effect powerfully projects the physician's image and reputation. Word of mouth has always been the best vehicle to market a medical practice.

How to Evaluate the Problem

- Review with the office manager the process and methods by which patients receive information about the doctor's practice.

- Is there a comprehensive policy and procedure manual that is kept current by staff members?

- Does an office brochure exist that affords useful information for patients? Is this brochure published on the practice's Web site where other information resources are offered?

- How much knowledge do all staff members possess about the practice and its operation to share with patients? Have they all read the policy and procedure manual?

- Is an office newsletter published to inform patients and to broadcast the distinguishing features of the medical practice?

- What information is contained in the telephone book listing?

- Are preprinted information sheets or pamphlets available to instruct targeted patient populations about the practice? Examples would be Medicare and Medicaid patients, pediatrics, selective HMO, and capitated populations.

- In what promotional and community activities is the practice involved?

- In what clinical or scientific research activities is the practice engaged, and what free publicity opportunities exist to gain exposure in the media?
- Does the practice have a computerized health maintenance program for automated health promotion activities?
- In the waiting room, do wall hangings and bulletin boards contain materials that provide practice information?

Cause for the Problem
- Too little time and effort devoted to informing the patient about the practice.
- Expense and effort required to produce printed materials, newsletters, and brochures.
- Incomplete staff knowledge about the practice, which often reflects a high staff turnover rate.
- The doctor may feel it is unnecessary or even inappropriate to showcase the practice.
- High patient turnover rates because of switching of insurance and doctor shopping.
- Costs related to a customized phone directory ad.
- Expense of a computerized information system and Web site to facilitate information sharing with patients.

Solutions
- Craft an office brochure, containing the full range of information about the practice, that can be used both for patient introduction to the practice and for marketing to potential patients. Include in the brochure thumbnail biographical sketches about the doctors. The brochure can be easily posted to a Web site.
- Encourage informal exchange of information between patients and the staff. Make certain the staff is fully aware and proud of the outstanding features of the practice. Their enthusiasm about the practice is contagious and motivates patients to seek more information.

- Collaboratively create a menu of pertinent practice information. Decide what items serve the interests of the patient. Brainstorm what means the practice can employ to reliably disseminate that information to all patients.

- Consider various promotional activities that mesh with the practice's strengths and services, such as health fairs, charity events, and sponsorship of seminars.

Costs

Brochures, phone book advertisements, Web sites, and tailored printed materials incur considerable expense, depending on how elaborate they are. Brochures can be simple and produced in large quantities at reasonable cost. Once the brochure format is in place, additional runs and minor changes are inexpensive.

A patient population that knows all about your practice is an asset that is cost effective to produce. Their positive testimonials are more compelling and build the practice's reputation. Patients ask fewer routine questions and initiate fewer nuisance calls. Finally, patients feel more connectivity with their doctor's practice.

Protect Patient Privacy

Patient's Perspective (figure A-6, page 114)

There are a number of privacy issues when the patient goes to see the doctor. Overall, the patient wants a shield against unnecessary exposure and release of confidential information. The experience of seeing the doctor is embarrassing to most patients and even humiliating to some.

Disclosure of psychiatric illness, sexually transmitted disease, injury, and other significant illnesses may pose a risk to some patients because of concerns about insurability, employability, legal issues, and possible social stigma. Patient expect encounters to be cloaked in confidentiality and respect for their dignity. Patients should be treated as if they were close relatives of the doctor. Privacy concerns, next to denial of illness, may be the most common cause for delay in seeking medical help. This issue often frustrates efforts to ensure continuity of care.

Figure A-6.

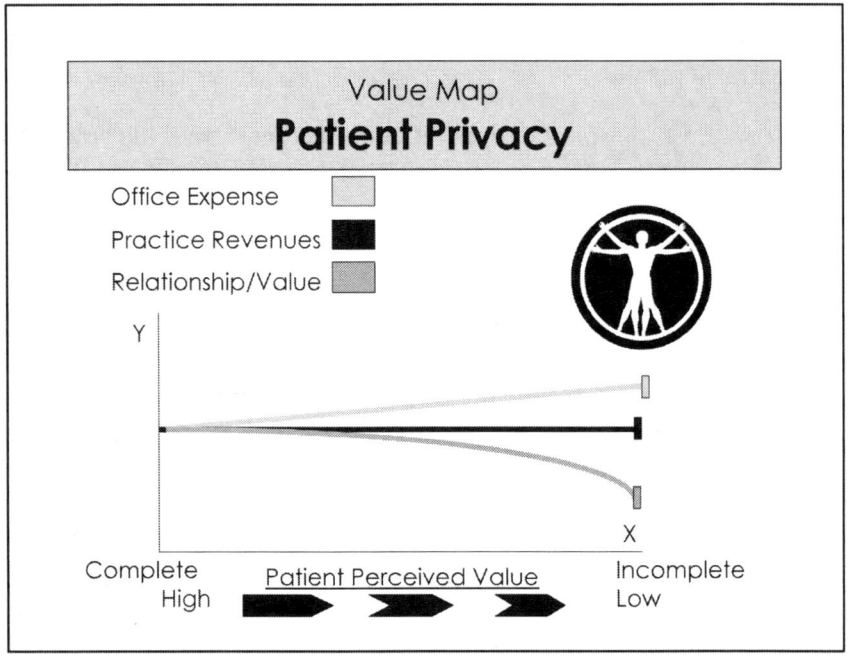

How to Identify the Problem

+ Read to outside persons the policy section in the office manual about confidentiality and information disclosure.

+ Observe movement of the chart and who makes entries during the patient encounter. Is the chart handled in such a way as to prevent other patients from reading it?

+ Are charts stored in a secure place? Is there a policy stating that the charts are always to remain in the offices of the medical practice?

+ Do front office personnel discuss patients in a way that can be heard in the waiting room by other patients?

+ Do office personnel project a professional demeanor and avoid discussing patient information outside the office.

+ Do dressing cubicles and screens exist in treatment rooms to prevent exposure during undressing and dressing? Is the patient offered an adequate gown, and are sheets used to minimize exposure during examination?

✦ Are chaperones used appropriately?

✦ Do the physicians avoid discussion of patient problems in the elevators and in public?

✦ Are patients counseled in the privacy of a consultation or examination room with closed doors?

✦ Are guidelines for public reporting of communicable diseases being followed?

Causes of the Problem

✦ An office environment that is too informal and casual.

✦ Insensitivity to diversity in personality traits. Individual patients interpret privacy differently.

✦ Failure to understand risk management issues in maintaining patient privacy.

✦ Lack of physician empathy.

✦ No written policy concerning confidentiality. If present, is it required reading for all employees?

✦ Insecure chart storage and transport.

Solutions

✦ Address modesty concerns by minimizing nudity in treatment areas.

✦ Encourage formality and professionalism in the office setting.

✦ Glass partition the reception desk and front work area from the waiting room.

✦ Ensure that charts are stored securely and not removed from the office.

✦ Have policy guidelines concerning release of information about patients.

Figure A-7.

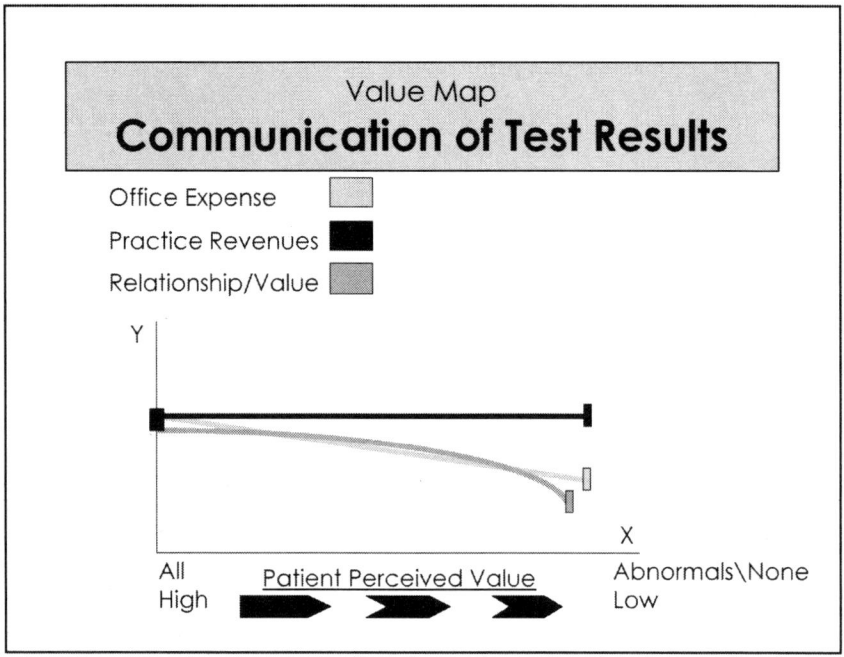

+ Foster physician and staff awareness of privacy concerns.

Costs

Costs are immaterial. Strict attention to privacy may occasionally slow patient flow, but this should not be significant if there is a sufficient number of treatment rooms in the office. Safeguards concerning information release do not affect office expense.

Communication of Test Results

Patient's Perspective (figure A-7, above)

Delays in sharing laboratory results create patient apprehension. Most patients want to be informed as soon as possible to relieve the worry that they have about an unsuspected illness or a condition that is worse than originally believed. The majority would like to know both normal and abnormal testing values and why they had to endure the bloodletting, ingestion of foreign substances, and indignity of body cavity probing.

Appendix A

To Identify the Problem

- Request that the office manager lead you through the process by which test results are reported to patients and communicated to the doctor. Is there a master list of ordered tests that are crossed off only after the results are received, and is the process automated electronically? When a test result is not received from a testing facility, is a call made to find out why? If the patient did not keep the appointment for testing, was he or she contacted to ask why and possibly to reschedule the testing?

- Are both normal and abnormal results reported to the patient? Who has the responsibility to monitor the reporting process?

- Is the result reported by phone, snail mail, fax, or e-mail, and how streamlined is the process?

- Do the physician and staff send personalized notes to the patient about office visit findings and laboratory results?

- When laboratory results are grossly abnormal, does the doctor call the patient to discuss the results and expeditiously schedule further studies if necessary?

- Are all critical or "panic" values immediately called to the attention of the doctor?

- Are test results placed in the chart or scanned into the EMR in a location where they can easily be retrieved?

- What steps are taken when a patient cannot be reached to relay an important result?

Causes of the Problem

- No process exists that records ordered tests, tracks the results, and reports them to the patient. No member of the office staff has the responsibility to monitor these activities.

- Complete reliance is placed on the patient to call for results. Often, practices tell patients that only abnormal results will be called when they are received. Frequently, the process precludes an adequate crosscheck to ensure that no result remains unreported.

- The testing facility may not be able to find the report, the patient may

Figure A-8.

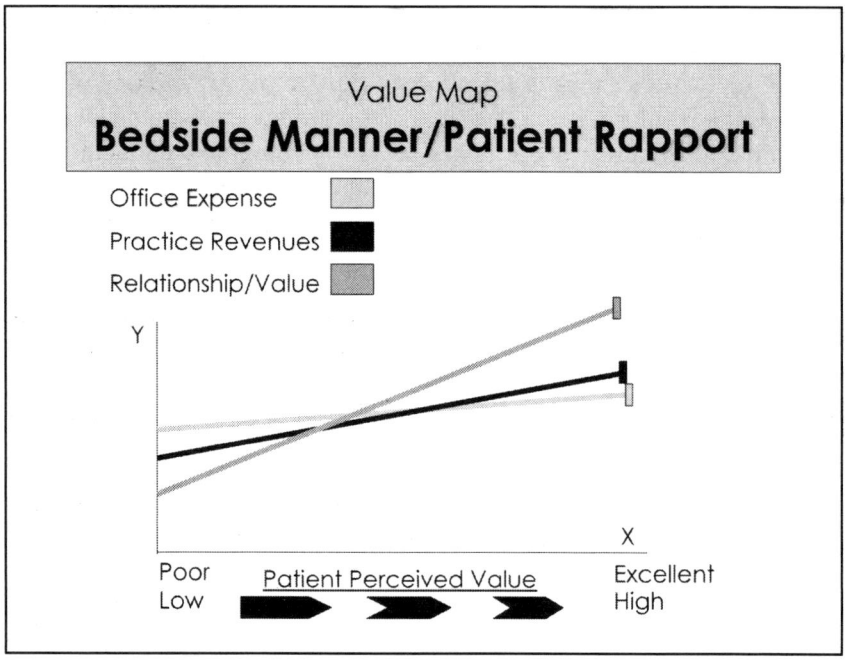

not have had the test performed, or the test may have to be repeated because of inconclusive results or faulty collection and transport.

Solutions

+ A standardized crosscheck process by which laboratory reports are consistently tracked, shared with the physician, and then communicated to the patient.

+ Fax and e-mail capability to expedite reception of reports and notification of the patient of normal results.

+ Communicate all abnormal test results and have the physician be the messenger if the test results have implications about treatment options or plans.

+ If the patient cannot be reached by phone but has an answering machine, leave a message to call the doctor but do not report laboratory results on an answering machine. To do so may violate confidentiality and cause the patient to miss the communication.

- If all efforts to reach the patient fail, send a letter advising the patient of the abnormal result and the need to contact the doctor's office.

Costs

If both normal and abnormal results are relayed, it can tie up additional time for someone in the office. Abnormal values should be communicated in a timely fashion. Reporting normal values delights the patient and helps to cement patient connectivity with the practice.

Bedside Manner and Face-to-Face Interaction with the Doctor

Patient's Perspective (figure A-8, page 118)

Nothing is more critical and more fundamental to the relationship than the social skills and caring of the doctor. Without linkage to physician empathy and concern, the patient experience is mechanical and disaffirming. Some physicians are naturally gifted with empathy and an ability to give of themselves. This supports a framework that fosters patient compliance and continuity of care. However, some doctors send signals that they are rushed and more focused on ending the encounter than on connecting with the patient. This dehumanizes the doctor/patient relationship and makes the patient feel like a number.

A good bedside manner and positive body language are essential to the practice of medicine. Medical school education often does not include adequate instruction in these critical skills that define the art of medicine. Caring or lack of caring may be intrinsic personality characteristics, but, fortunately, key behaviors—interviewing skills, a good bedside manner, ability to communicate effectively, and positive body language—are disciplines that can be taught and mastered by all physicians. Most studies show that the length of time spent in the patient encounter is of less importance to patient satisfaction than the quality of the time spent.

To Identify the Problem

- Patient satisfaction surveys that ask if the physician seemed rushed and solicit a description of the quality of the face-to-face interview with the physician. Did the physician project warmth and have good communication skills and an engaging personality?

- ✦ Question the medical assistant about the doctor's relationship with patients. What criticisms do patients express?
- ✦ Ask front office personnel about the feedback they receive from patients and their families as they prepare to exit the office.

Causes of the Problem

- ✦ A physician who chronically feels rushed and pushes patient flow.
- ✦ A physician who does not enjoy patient contact and gives the impression that he or she does not wish to fully engage in the close relationships that are a part of clinical practice.
- ✦ Lack of empathy and caring that produces a failure to understand the patient's emotional support needs.
- ✦ An impaired physician with emotional problems.
- ✦ Physician "burn-out."
- ✦ Cultural differences between doctor and patient.
- ✦ Often, physicians have little insight as to the quality of their bedside manner and body language. Some have difficulty with personal relationships and build defenses that shield the physician from patient feedback and the flexibility to sharpen their "people skills."

Solutions

- ✦ If the physician is receptive to constructive criticism, he or she can learn improved social and communication skills, plus reinforcing of body language.
- ✦ Training in psychology to improve understanding of the emotional underpinnings of the patient in the physician encounters.
- ✦ Appointment scheduling that does not chronically rush the physician and that provides unhurried time for the physician to connect with the patient. This enables the physician to answer questions and address the full range of patient concerns.
- ✦ Instruction of office personnel to "fill in the gaps" left when the doctor does not provide the emotional support or adequate instructions expected by the patient.

- Dissemination of biographical information about the physician to the patient to act as an entry point for sharing common interests between the patient and the doctor. This puts a "human face" on the doctor.

- Counseling exercises that enhance awareness that a confidant, cheerful, and optimistic attitude promotes a close relationship and improves compliance.

- Measure patient satisfaction scores on questions about the physician's demeanor and behavior, and set goals for improving those scores.

- Teach the physician that a participatory, interactive style of office management can build his or her reputation and respect with the office staff. A testimonial from the employee who works for the "best doctor in town" is a powerful message that builds image and trust and adds to the positive perception of the physician's bedside manner.

- Learn to paraphrase big medical terms in language the patient understands.

Costs

A little extra high-quality time goes a long way toward solidifying the doctor/patient relationship and translates into patient loyalty, keeping of appointments, and referral of friends. Retention of loyal patients provides lower transaction costs than acquiring new patients. When viewed from the lifetime of revenues generated by a loyal patient base, it can be seen that a good relationship and bedside manner pay huge continuing dividends.

Uncomfortable or Unappealing Office

Patient's Perspective (figure A-9, page 122)

The ambience and appearance of the office are a direct reflection of the physician. Descriptors of an office such as dirty, cluttered, outdated, small, and poorly decorated send a negative message to the patient about the way the doctor practices and conducts his or her professional life.

To Identify the Problem

- What do offices of competing practices look like?

- What member of the staff has the responsibility for tidying, decorating, and maintaining the front and back office?

Figure A-9.

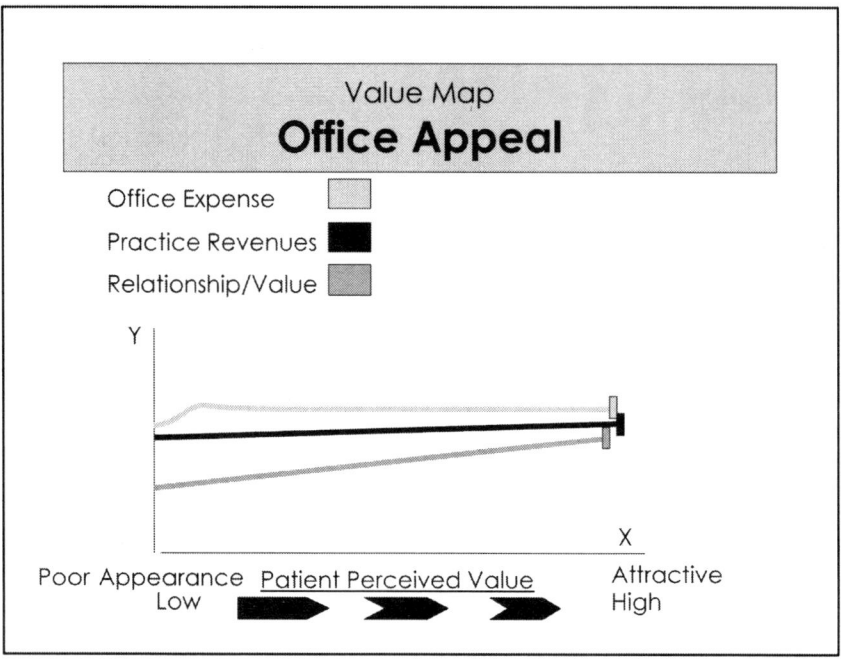

- ✦ Visualize what could be done to improve the atmosphere and the ambience of the office.

- ✦ What do the office manager and physician's spouses think of the physical design and furnishings of the office?

- ✦ On patient satisfaction surveys, what criticisms have patients had concerning the physical appearance of the office?

Causes of the Problem

- ✦ A cleaning service that does only perfunctory cleaning, and a building manager who provides inadequate maintenance.

- ✦ My office has looked like this for two decades. Why change now?

- ✦ The doctor does not want to invest money to redecorate and renovate the office and/or is convinced that the office environment is of secondary importance.

- The practice rented the cheapest suite available, with minimum square footage.

- A physical layout that allows patients to see the clutter in the business office.

- Lack of covered or concealed storage space, and storage of obsolete or redundant equipment in hallways and treatment rooms.

- No dedicated physician consultation rooms, requiring conferences with patients and families to be held in treatment rooms that appear sterile and cold.

- An office staff that is oblivious to the problem and does not view it as its responsibility to maintain the appearance of the office.

Solutions

- Get outside impartial opinions about the ambiance of the office.

- Assign ownership of the appearance of the office to the office manager or another member of the staff.

- Enlist the help of spouses to make the office have the refinements of home.

- Evaluate the quality of the housekeeping service, and insist that the building owners paint and redecorate when needed.

Costs

Your office décor should be as carefully planned as that of your home. Its image in the eyes of the patient is a reflection of your image. Renovation requires a one-time fixed cost but can be enjoyed by your staff and patients for many years. If the owner of your building does not maintain it, move to another location.

Managing the Phone (figure A-10, page 124)

Patient's Perspective

The phone is an interface with all of your customers—patients, suppliers, referring doctors, and so on. If your phone door is configured to limit calls, it causes irritation and customer dissatisfaction. Automated systems with several levels of options often confuse and put off patients

Figure A-10.

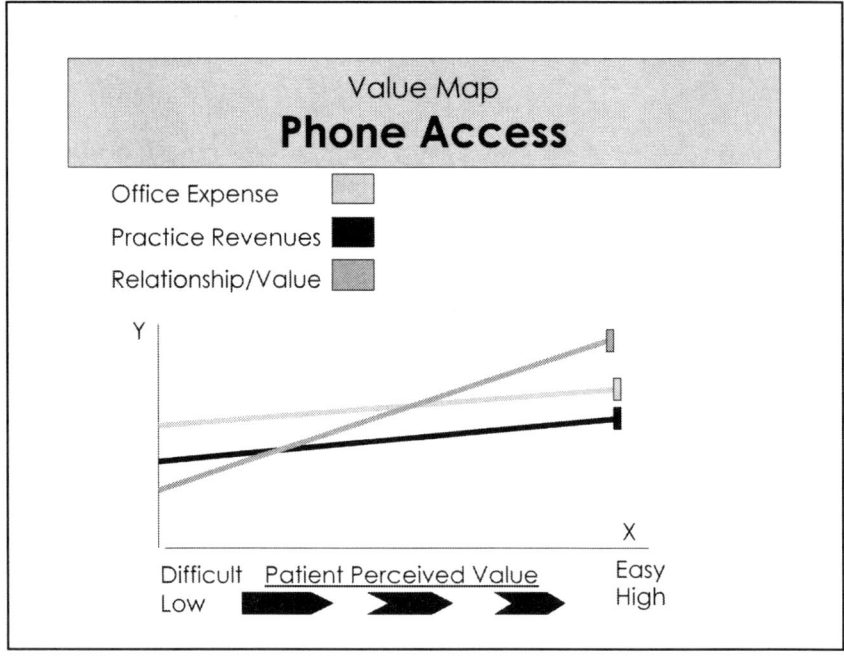

who wish to speak to a human. Endless busy signals waste patient time, produce patient frustration and anger, result in legitimate important calls' being unanswered, and drive patients to seek other alternatives. A phone call usually consumes a fixed amount of time whenever it is answered. Why postpone it?

Patients expect to receive courteous service over the phone. The telephone welcome is a direct reflection of the office culture.

To Identify the Problem

✦ Ask the phone company to assess the "busy rate" percentage and the adequacy of the number of incoming lines.

✦ Inquire about your "phone door" in patient satisfaction surveys.

✦ Phone calls are the bane of an office staff's existence; what tactics have been employed to control the number of incoming calls?

- Does the office staff sign off the phone during the lunch break for its convenience and not that of persons trying to reach the doctor?
- Do employees sign out to the answering service before office hours are concluded?
- Is there a private line for important incoming and outgoing calls?
- What is the office process for filtering and sorting calls to the doctor, billing specialist, and back office?
- Review the yellow page phone listing. Is it easily found in bold print, and does it provide information about the practice.
- Is the staff trained in phone etiquette and answering techniques?
- What strategies, such as fax and e-mail, has the practice used to decrease phone usage?

Solutions

- The telephone is the portal for your business; ensure that you have an adequate number of lines and sufficient personnel to answer the phone during peak phone hours.
- Target phone pick-up within four rings.
- Coordinate with the office staff the process that manages the phone.
- Keep the phone door open throughout office hours.
- Target short holding times for incoming calls. Make certain your office representative identifies who is calling before placing them on hold.
- Encourage patients to make non-urgent calls to the practice during low-volume periods.
- Standardize the opening phone answering greeting to project warmth and willingness to help.
- Develop a format and filtering process for directing calls to the appropriate party.
- Have a policy about personal phone calls.

- When a patient is placed on hold, someone should get back to him or her at least every 30 seconds with the status of the call.

- Creatively use electronic e-mail and fax, plus look at e-commerce solutions to decrease the volume of incoming and outgoing calls. Transactions such as receiving and sending lab results, checking eligibility, obtaining preauthorizations, scheduling appointments and tests, and receiving and sending patient information can be automated to bypass phone communication. This permits these activities to be performed at the convenience of the staff.

Costs

Improved phone service may incur some increase in monthly phone charges and stress the office personnel during peak hours, such as Monday mornings and lunchtime. However, these are not critical considerations when balanced against the capture of all calls and improved patient service and access. All medical practices need to look at the frontier of electronic information technology that will enable efficient information transfer and circumvent the labor-intensive telephone. Long-term, state-of-the-art information technology will decrease costs and increase productivity.

Untimely Correspondence Response

Patient's Perspective (figure A-11, page 127)

Many patients and other parties need information from your practice—the Bureau of Workman's Compensation, lawyers in liability and injury cases, insurance companies, employers, hospitals, doctors who have received referrals from your practice, other physicians, relatives, unemployment agencies, case managers, and so on. The response time and adequacy of information transfer reflects on the efficiency of your practice. Postponing or procrastination does not decrease the amount of time it takes to fill out a form or dictate a letter. The perception of your practice from these individuals and agencies rests with your prompt attention.

To Identify the Problem

- Ask the office manager what the average delay is in answering correspondence? How many second and third requests are received?

Figure A-11.

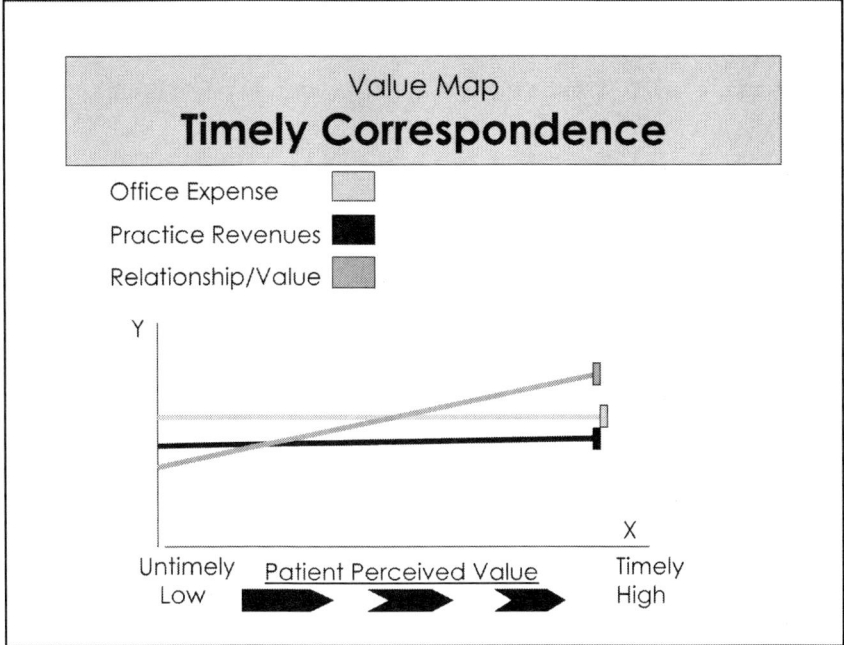

- ✦ Look on the physician's desk; if he or she is behind, you will easily identify a stack of papers relating to requests for information.
- ✦ Ask the billing specialist about delays in sending requested information to insurance companies.

Causes of the Problem:

- ✦ Embedded bad habits.
- ✦ Inadequate or lack of a system that transcribes dictation and/or an information system that does not automate the process.
- ✦ Physician indifference, inadequate time, or sheer procrastination.
- ✦ Paper files or records can't be found.

Solutions

- ✦ Address the physician's behavior and attitudes.

- ✦ Standardize the process by which requests for information are received and fulfilled. Ensure that requests do not get buried and intermingled with piles of other miscellaneous paper materials.
- ✦ Delegate selected reporting duties to the staff, to be sent out over the physician's signature.
- ✦ Procure transcription equipment and generate correspondence in house.
- ✦ Use electronic technology to efficiently support the process.

Costs

There is no increase in office expense. However, it improves the image and reputation of the practice when correspondence receives prompt attention.

Appendix B
Health Maintenance Software: An Essential Component

Health maintenance programs focus on four categories of activity: counseling, screening evaluation, immunizations, and chemoprophylaxis regimens for patients before they develop clinical evidence of disease.

To attempt a health maintenance program without an information technology infrastructure is virtually impossible. There is too much information and tracking to manage with a paper system. Most health maintenance software programs interface with or are a part of the EMR. Some stand-alone programs exist, but they introduce inefficiency because of the need for double data entry.

In general, three types of applications exist in health maintenance programs.

✦ **Health risk appraisal:** Health risk assessment (HRA) software is available from many vendors. These interactive programs assist in identifying risk factors, assigning a patient risk score, and suggesting items to track.

✦ Development of risk-related health maintenance protocols that individual practices can develop on the basis of the characteristics of the practice

- ✦ Health maintenance tracking with a tickler function that generates "to do" lists and reminders.

Creating a health maintenance program is best accomplished through collaboration with all staff members. This assists in embedding the concepts in the practice culture and helps to cement it as an ongoing commitment.

Appendix C
Dollars and Cents of an EMR

Going beyond conventional practice management systems, the EMR has been acknowledged by the medical community as a logical extension of technology into clinic management. Current statistics reveal that 26 percent of physician practices cite an immediate need for patient record computerization and 72 percent project a need for electronic patient record keeping within five years.

A Case Scenario

Most clients have experienced a positive return on investment. The following data detail the savings in overhead expense achieved by the North Fulton Family Medicine practice in Alpharetta, Georgia, using the HealthMatics EMR offered by A4 Health Systems. In response to rapid expansion, this group began strategic planning in 1996. The practice profile includes two office locations and full activation of the EMR, with a paperless office beginning on December 17, 1998. The practice has four physician associates and 12 front office and six back office professional personnel to cover both office locations. The EMR program is used in approximately 100 patient encounters per day.

Time and Labor for Chart Management before and after Introduction of EMR System

	Minutes/Day Before	Minutes/Day After
Chart Handling	625	25
Creating New paper Charts	190	0
Missing Chart Search	330	0

Results: The practice eliminated three of its four full-time file clerks, for a savings of approximately $70,000 per year.

Transcription Expense

	Minutes/Day Before	Minutes/Day After
Transcription expense	705	0
Referral letter transcription expense	180	0

Results: The practice eliminated two full-time transcriptionists plus some outsourcing costs, for a savings of approximately $142,000 per year.

Laboratory Result Handling Costs

	Minutes/Day Before	Minutes/Day After
Laboratory log and reporting	570	0

Results: Savings of $31,000 per year.

Chart Supply Costs

Supply Costs/Year Before	Supply costs/Year After
$24,480	0

Results: Elimination of the expense of pre-printed forms and charting materials. Additionally, the practice no longer needed to transport charts or waste space with chart storage.

In summary, the practice saved approximately 44 staff hours per day or 11,968 hours per year. This equated to $253,978 dollars per year in

Appendix C
Dollars and Cents of an EMR

Going beyond conventional practice management systems, the EMR has been acknowledged by the medical community as a logical extension of technology into clinic management. Current statistics reveal that 26 percent of physician practices cite an immediate need for patient record computerization and 72 percent project a need for electronic patient record keeping within five years.

A Case Scenario

Most clients have experienced a positive return on investment. The following data detail the savings in overhead expense achieved by the North Fulton Family Medicine practice in Alpharetta, Georgia, using the HealthMatics EMR offered by A4 Health Systems. In response to rapid expansion, this group began strategic planning in 1996. The practice profile includes two office locations and full activation of the EMR, with a paperless office beginning on December 17, 1998. The practice has four physician associates and 12 front office and six back office professional personnel to cover both office locations. The EMR program is used in approximately 100 patient encounters per day.

Time and Labor for Chart Management before and after Introduction of EMR System

	Minutes/Day Before	Minutes/Day After
Chart Handling	625	25
Creating New paper Charts	190	0
Missing Chart Search	330	0

Results: The practice eliminated three of its four full-time file clerks, for a savings of approximately $70,000 per year.

Transcription Expense

	Minutes/Day Before	Minutes/Day After
Transcription expense	705	0
Referral letter transcription expense	180	0

Results: The practice eliminated two full-time transcriptionists plus some outsourcing costs, for a savings of approximately $142,000 per year.

Laboratory Result Handling Costs

	Minutes/Day Before	Minutes/Day After
Laboratory log and reporting	570	0

Results: Savings of $31,000 per year.

Chart Supply Costs

Supply Costs/Year Before	Supply costs/Year After
$24,480	0

Results: Elimination of the expense of pre-printed forms and charting materials. Additionally, the practice no longer needed to transport charts or waste space with chart storage.

In summary, the practice saved approximately 44 staff hours per day or 11,968 hours per year. This equated to $253,978 dollars per year in office expense just on the documented functions of chart pulls, new patient chart generation, missing chart searches, transcription, lab result handling, referral letters, and medical chart supplies. This example clearly shows the potential to recapture the initial investment costs for electronic automation within a short time.

Moreover, the majority of medical practices generate additional revenues from the coding application provided by most EMR programs. In a small sample, roughly 15 percent of patient encounters were appropriately and accurately up-coded; thus producing about $10,000 of billed charges per physician per year.

Related Books

Albrecht, K. *The Only Thing that Matters*. New York, N.Y.: Harper Business Books, 1992.

Annis, E. 1993. *Code Blue: Health Care in Crisis*. Washington, D.C.: Regnery Gateway, 1993.

Brown, S., and others. 1993. *Patient Satisfaction Pays*. Gaithersburg, Md.: Aspen Publishers, 1993.

Covey, S. *The 7 Habits of Highly Effective People*. New York, N.Y.: Simon and Schuster, 1989.

Gale, B. *Managing Customer Value: Creating Quality and Service that Customers Can See*. New York, N.Y.: Free Press, 1994.

Goldstein, D. *E-Healthcare: Harness the Power of Internet E-Commerce & E-Care*. Gaithersburg, Md.: Aspen Publishers, 2000.

Goleman, D. *Working with Emotional Intelligence*. New York, N.Y.: Bantam Books, 1998.

Herzlinger, R. *Market-Driven Health Care*. Cambridge, Mass.: Perseus, 1997.

Hesselbein, F., and others, Editors. *The Leader of the Future*. San Francisco, Calif.: Jossey-BAss, 1996.

Landholt, T. *Automating the Medical Record*. Chicago, Ill.: American Medical Association, 1999.

Lucas, H. *Information Technology and the Productivity Paradox: Assessing the Value of Investing in IT*. New York, N.Y.: Oxford University Press, 1999.

Lundberg, G. *Severed Trust: Why American Medicine Hasn't Been Fixed*. New York, N.Y.: Basic Books, 2000.

Morreim, E. *Balancing Act: The New Medical Ethics of Medicine's New Economics*. Washington, D.C.: Georgetown University Press, 1995.

Reichheld, F. 1996. *The Loyalty Effect: The Hidden Force behind Growth, Profits, and Lasting Value.* Boston, Mass.: Harvard Business School Press, 1996.

Sherman, S. 1999. *Total Customer Satisfaction: A Comprehensive Approach for Health Care Providers.* San Francisco: Jossey-Bass, 1999.

Whiteley, R., and Hessan, D. Customer Centered Growth: *Five Proven Strategies for Building Competitive Advantage.* Cambridge, Mass.: Perseus, 1996.

Wilkerson, J., and others. *Competitive Managed Care: The Emerging Health Care System.* San Francisco, Calif.: Jossey-Bass, 1997.

Woolf, S., and others. *Health Promotion and Disease Prevention in Clinical Practice.* Baltimore, Md.: Williams and Wilkins, 1996.

We've Made Your Mouse Mighty!

Now, at the click of a mouse, you can gain access to the latest thinking on critical issues in medical management. All of it comes to you in *Click*, the American College of Physician Executives' on-line journal for physician executives. You can access *Click* at www.acpe.org/click.

- In-depth articles that explore the leading edge of medical management issues and trends.

- Feedback mechanism for comments on an article or on your efforts in the area covered by an article.

- Additional resources on the topic covered by an article.

- Access to comments from reviewers and readers of the article.

Don't take our word for it. The best way to experience this new publishing venture is to see it first-hand. Take your mouse on a visit to *Click*.

You May Have Paid Too Much for This Book

Members of the American College of Physician Executives receive discounts and special prices on all of our educational and informational products.

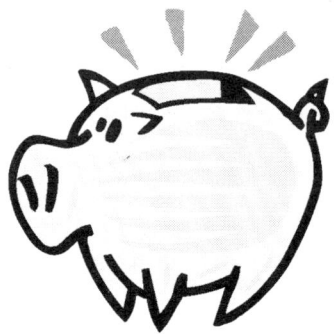

On a single item, that may not seem like much, but a few books and attendance at an educational program can sometimes recover an entire year's membership dues.

That is only one of many reasons for joining the College, of course. Many of our programs are offered only to members. The Graduate Program in Medical Management, whereby completion of College educational programs in the first step to a master's degree in medical management from a prestigious university, is a prime example.

The best reason for joining the College is the many opportunities to network with other physicians who have opted for management careers. In a variety of formal and informal programs, the College encourages and promotes the concept of networking and group discussion. The addition of Internet services has made networking an easy and compelling method of growing a management career.

Give us a call at **800/562-8088**
or drop by our Web site **(www.acpe.org)**
to learn more about the advantages of membership in ACPE.